JACOB CRAIG

INSPIRING
LEADERS

— in —

Health
&
Fitness

Vol. 1

THE ULTIMATE GUIDE
TO BUILDING A BETTER YOU

INSPIRING LEADERS IN HEALTH & FITNESS
THE ULTIMATE GUIDE TO BUILDING A BETTER YOU
VOL. 1
FIRST EDITION
By Jacob Craig (www.inspiringleaderscollective.com)
Copyright © 2021 Jacob Marchand, Inspiring Leaders Collective

This book is a general educational health-related information product and is intended for healthy adults age 18 or over.
This book is solely for information and educational purposes and does not constitute medical advice. Please consult a medical or health professional before you begin any exercise, nutrition, or supplementation program or if you have questions about your health. There may be risks associated with participating in activities or using products mentioned in this book for people in poor health or with preexisting physical or mental health conditions. Because these risks exist, you should not use the products or participate in the activities described in this book if you are in poor health or if you have a preexisting mental or physical health condition. If you choose to participate in these activities, you do so knowingly and voluntarily of your own free will and accord, assuming all risks associated with these activities. Specific results mentioned in this book should be considered extraordinary, and there are no "typical" results. Because individuals differ, results will differ.

Cover designed by Damonza (*www.damonza.com*)
Edited by Olayiwola Janet Oluwatobiloba
Portraits done by Natalya Kopylova
Published by Inspiring Leaders Collective (*www.inspiringleaderscollective.com*)

ISBN: 978-1-7363781-0-6 Print
ISBN: 978-1-7363781-1-3 Ebook

*To Taylor, for supporting me through
the researching, writing, and publishing process.*

*And to my parents, for being dedicated, hard workers
and setting such a great example for what I aspire to be.*

CONTENTS

FOREWORD

The path to obtaining optimal health, fitness, and wellness can often be confusing and contradictory. It can be downright tiring, especially when you're trying to keep up with so many popular trends. It can even get depressing if you've listened to expert health tips on social media and find yourself unable to keep up with what you should and shouldn't do. But, honestly, it shouldn't be that hard to find the right information on how to achieve your health and fitness goals.

Most health, wellness, and nutrition experts in their field have tried-and-proven tips that work based on science, experiments, and experience. However, a common problem most of us have is that we are overloaded with information from many sources, making it hard to focus and isolate the most important health and wellness tips to keep us focused on our own path.

Inspiring Leaders in Health & Fitness is a collection of actionable tips, ideas, concepts, and thoughts from leading experts in the health and wellness field including nutritionists, strength and conditioning coaches, and physical therapists. Each chapter focuses on one guru and discusses their path to greatness as well their groundbreaking rise to becoming well-respected members of the health and fitness community. Their chapters discuss their scientifically-based principles and strategies for keeping us safe and healthy. And for balance, each chapter discusses contradicting thoughts and ideologies as well as shared thoughts between all experts. The knowledge from the experts shared in this book is applicable to anyone who is interested in learning how to become their own top-notch health or fitness coach, or even someone who needs off-classroom health and wellness pointers, either for personal reasons, school, work, or business.

Optimal health is a combination of nutrition and physical activity, including strength and conditioning. It also involves a coordinated mind and soul, and the various experts in this book bring this concept to life. Though there are tons of similarities between what each expert says and believes, there are also nuances that make them stand apart, even controversies and conflicts, making each chapter worth reading and learning from. Knowing that total fitness involves more than just the physical body makes it easier to start on a well-balanced wellness journey based on your personal goals.

For students who are searching for more knowledge for academic or personal goals, the thoughts and ideas contained within *Inspiring Leaders in Health & Fitness*, will complement and even add to what you learn in the classroom. For instance, if you're a physical therapy student, the skills shared by the expert physical therapist with years of experience will be beneficial in learning other ways to do things better. If you are a nutrition student striving for more knowledge, the expert nutritionists discussed here have years of experience that would offer significant insights that you might not easily find in one place. Or if you are an exercise student, the many valuable sections on exercise, diet, fitness, muscle-building, and so many more will put you ahead of the curve as you will pick up several ideas that you might never have had access to otherwise. Learning from experts in the industry will make you a significantly better student and applying their relatively balanced approach to health and fitness will make you a better athlete with advanced nutrition skills.

Inspiring Leaders in Health & Fitness also serves as a great research tool for writers in the health, fitness, and nutrition field since the experts discussed within the book were selected over a two-year period of rigorous research and analysis. Many of them are authors whose books have also been referenced. Their published books, along with *Inspiring Leaders in Health & Fitness*, will not only serve as resource for anyone passionate about reading and writing health and wellness books, but is also ideal for someone who simply wants to take their personal fitness goals to the next level.

The collection of knowledge from the experts in *Inspiring Leaders in Health & Fitness, Vol 1* includes some of the best insights in the industry and their background and works in the industry reflect hundreds of years of experience, distilled into one book. This book will show you how to live longer, stronger, healthier, and happier. There are so many connections between all parts of fitness and wellness and knowing how to use them, through the ideas presented in here, is a great way to advance your personal health and fitness journey.

Shawn Stevenson, the first health and nutrition expert analyzed in this book, focuses not only on general health and nutrition but also highlights the importance of sleep to our overall health and wellbeing. As a sleep expert and someone who has researched extensively on the benefits of sleep in reversing chronic diseases as well as in slowing the progress of many diseases, Shawn has great hacks on how to get more quality sleep which ultimately leads to better health and fitness. His biography also discusses the importance of continuously moving the body, something that we are all too guilty of not doing. As a nutritionist, he is able to offer insights on how nutrition, sleep, and movement interplay for a healthier life. If you are someone who is sleep-deprived like most of us are, or someone struggling with getting better sleep, his insights on sleep and overall wellness will be beneficial to getting you to a better and healthier place.

For those of us who live a plant-powered life, want to adapt a plant-based diet, or struggle with autoimmune diseases with limited treatment success, the section on **Dr. Gundry**, a heart surgeon, physician and a dietician who focuses on a plant-based diet, is a great start for learning the proper science and benefits of a plant-based diet on our overall health. Dr. Gundry is also fondly known as "The Fixer" in the medical world because his methods have helped people lose weight and cure certain chronic diseases. His chapter offers tips that are not only critical to longevity, but also important for anyone wishing to remain healthy and fit as they age. Plant-powered diets are extremely popular and Dr. Gundry's expertise will guide you towards being more knowledgeable about how best to make plants work for your body to achieve your health and fitness goals.

Ben Greenfield, an expert physical fitness coach and trainer, ex-bodybuilder, speaker on health and wellness, and author, offers insights on several health topics including performance and recovery, High Intensity Interval Training (HIIT), and Cold Thermogenesis. For people who wonder how athletic performance is connected to recovery, Ben's chapter is a great start to learn about how to support the body's performance through faster recovery. As a biohacker, he often experiments on ways to increase the efficiency of our body through technology. Ben is also dedicated to nutrition, lifestyle, and sleep, and through his views, you will learn unique hacks for more quality longevity based on the principles of nutrition, brain health, sleep, and fitness.

Diet and sleep are very important for healthy living and are major components to our health and fitness but strength and conditioning also plays an important role in our overall fitness. For anyone wanting to build muscle in a way that is easy yet efficient, **Michael Matthews**, a top strength and conditioning coach as well as author of many popular books including books on building muscle the right way, is the right person to listen and learn from. The chapter dedicated to his work has insights on how to get leaner and stronger amongst many other tips. For those interested in the science behind dietary supplements and how they work, Michael is also an expert in dietary supplements and offers great insights on how to safely incorporate supplements into your health and fitness routine.

If you've ever wanted the advice of a physician and nutritionist who has worked with top professional athletes and has created a renowned nutritional program, **Dr. Cate Shanahan** should be your go-to person. Many of us know how to eat right and what to avoid but an expert like Dr. Cate goes into microdetails of nutrition including the science behind simple things like oils and sugars, and how and why fresh foods should be our priority. Her expertise is backed by clear research and field experience. If you are dedicated to good nutrition but want to know exactly why you should avoid certain foods, her portion of the book has fresh insights that can help you be more successful in your journey to better health through proper nutrition. And if you are a nutrition student wanting to learn more about the principles of good nutrition, her portion of the book will take you outside the box but with solid scientific backing.

What about physical therapy? Is it important to health and fitness? Very much so! Learning how to treat your body kindly during an intense workout while using the proper mechanics of your body to your advantage amongst so many other things is something renewed athlete, physical therapist, and strength and conditioning coach **Kelly Starrett** will show you in the chapter dedicated to his work. Also, fans of the popular CrossFit program will be glad to know that Kelly is deeply connected to the CrossFit community as former owner of a CrossFit gym. For anyone who wants to learn how to train and condition safer and more efficiently, Kelly's chapter offers expertise on using the principles of physical therapy for safer training and conditioning of the body.

Even though there are different schools of thoughts on the best path to health and fitness, reading and adopting the research, ideas, thoughts, and experiences from some of the best in the field as presented in *Inspiring Leaders in Health & Fitness*, is a great start for athletes and health-conscious individuals interested in the art and science of better fitness and nutrition.

Myrah Summers
Medical Professional/Writer
Certified by the American Medical Writers Association

AUTHOR'S PREFACE

Truth be told, the reason that I started the process of writing this book was really for myself. I was working out regularly (every other day) with a decent variety of exercises and I knew my diet needed improvement but I didn't think it was that bad at the time. Nonetheless, I had been doing that for a year or so with about 20 pounds of fat I wanted to lose and I was only able to lose about 5.

My goal was to lose that weight and then try to build as much muscle as I could. I honestly had no idea what I was doing. I never did contact sports growing up so the only weight training experience I'd gotten was a couple gym classes in high school that took place in a room with nice equipment and a few trips to the gym with my family or college buddies.

So one day, I started listening to advice from certain influencers that I follow. I started reading books, looking at cookbooks that pushed me towards eating whole, natural foods rather than processed foods, and researching people in the health and fitness space that had earned respect from others and had an enormous following of people they've helped through their advice and programs.

As I was doing this research, I realized just how much information was out there. I thought that if I made it a goal to research twelve experts with different backgrounds over a twelve-month timeframe, I would be able to learn a whole lot and find both an exercise plan and diet plan that works for me.

To really commit to this and to push this idea further, I decided to write about what I was researching. This would not only help me learn the information more (we all know writing something down helps commit it to memory) but I figured there are many people who could use this valuable information in their lives as well and if my writing only helps one person change their lives for the better, it is all worth it.

You'll quickly realize that this book is not on twelve experts as I originally planned. Hence why this is "*Vol. 1.*" Many of these experts had too much content to cover in 1 month's time so I would spend 2-3 months per expert instead. I not only researched their free content like podcasts, blog posts, and YouTube videos but paid content as well like their books and programs.

The amount of content that I examined from each of these individuals adds up to hundreds of hours of listening, watching, and reading per. In each biography, I share how each of them got the platform that they have now as well as *each* and *every* tip and trick that I found helpful for me or I thought is worth sharing with the general public who are interested in improving their health and fitness.

You'll find that I attempted to research all different backgrounds, from nutrition to strength and conditioning to physical therapy. Although all of these experts are known to be reputable and are generally well-respected, my intent is not for you to follow *all* of their advice. In fact, that is not possible. Just as much as they share beliefs, they contradict each other and I do my best to reiterate these points at the end of each expert's biography. From there, you can choose what diet and exercise programs work best for you and suit your goals.

There are two ways to go about reading *Inspiring Leaders in Health & Fitness*:

1. You can simply read start to finish. You'll read every biography in order and the "Shared Thoughts" and "Contradicting Thoughts" sections at the end of each biography may make more sense because they will relate the expert you just learned about to those discussed prior.
2. You can go to the Brief Leader Bios, read each expert's bio, and choose who interests you most and start with their biography. Then,

after you finish reading their biography, go back to the Brief Leader Bios and choose the next expert until you've read all six. Lastly, move on to the Conclusion and read in order from there.

While each expert is worth knowing and will have valuable tips, you may read this book and only find one or two that you decide to follow. Honestly, that's fantastic because each of these individuals has enough content and enough inspiration to make a real positive change in your life.

I hope that you enjoy reading this book and if you have any questions or comments along the way, you can always reach me at jake@inspringleaderscollective.com. I personally answer all of my emails and I greatly appreciate any and all feedback, good or bad, so that I can improve and the following edition can be corrected if need be.

Now that you have a good sense of what this book is about, why I decided to write it, and how it could benefit you, let's get started!

FREE BONUS MATERIALS (GUIDES, VIDEOS, ARTICLES, AND MORE!)

You'll notice as you're reading this book the amount of research done before writing. While the biographies contained herein describe the experts that I pay attention to along with an overview of their content and how they've built the platform and reputation that they have today, there is more to be seen behind the scenes.

First, this book will be the first of a series through **www.InspiringLeadersCollective.com**.

Second, as I do my ongoing research, I also share my findings through articles on my personal blog, **www.TwelvePaths.com**. I share reviews on books, programs, podcasts, and supplements as well as articles that compare and contrast tips from a variety of experts on specific topics.

If you subscribe to my newsletter on **www.TwelvePaths.com**, you will not only get news about articles, book releases, and website updates, but you will immediately receive two free PDF Guides that I've created: "Your Guide to Nutrition & Fitness" and "Your Guide on How to Get & Stay Inspired."

Third, I have started a YouTube Channel, **www.youtube.com/ inspiringleaderscollective**, where I share more content including informative interviews and content similar to what is found on my personal blog.

Last, if you every have any questions or comments, you can always email me at **jake@inspiringleaderscollective.com**. I will do my best to assist you or point you in the right direction, no matter what question you have related to my content.

All of this content is proudly completed by myself (aside from editors, designers, and other support through the process).

BRIEF LEADER BIOS

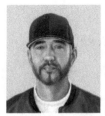 **Shawn Stevenson**, aka "The Sleep Expert," is the bestselling author of *Sleep Smarter* and founder of the popular health and wellness podcast, *The Model Health Show*, which has been at the top of the charts since its start in 2013.

Through his platform, he has worked to help thousands of people to reach their health and wellness goals. He has articles, podcasts, and even masterclasses on specific topics such as: sleep, fat loss, relationships, water, sugar, blood pressure, and more. His work has been featured in many popular outlets including ESPN, *Forbes, The Dr. Oz Show, Men's Health, Women's Health, The Huffington Post*, FOX, and more.

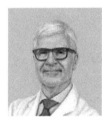 **Dr. Steven Gundry**, aka "The Fixer," is a former heart surgeon turned dietitian. He is the New York Times bestselling author of *The Plant Paradox, The Longevity Paradox*, as well as two other books. He is also a YouTuber, blogger, and podcaster through his website, *DrGundry.com*.

His plant-based approach to fixing gut health has helped thousands lose weight and/or overcome health issues such as: heart disease, Lupus, Crohn's Disease, Rheumatoid Arthritis, stage 3 & 4 cancers, and more. His work has been featured in many popular outlets including *The Dr. Oz Show*, NPR, FOX, GQ, ABC, and People.

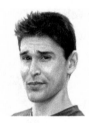 **Ben Greenfield** is an author of over a dozen books, including his New York Times bestsellers *Beyond Training* and *Boundless*. He is a former top traithlete and ex-bodybuilder (amongst many other things) who also has a popular website and podcast, *Ben Greenfield Fitness*, and is the founder of Kion.

Through his books, podcast, and virtual coaching, he has helped thousands of high-performing athletes and CEOs be at the top of their game mentally and physically. His work has been featured in many popular outlets including WebMD, FOX, *The Joe Rogan Experience, The Huffington Post*, NBC, and CBS.

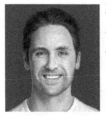

Michael Matthews is a bestselling fitness author of *Bigger Leaner Stronger*, *Thinner Leaner Stronger*, and *The Shredded Chef*, as well the founder of Legion Athletics.

His simple and science-based approach to building muscle, losing fat, and getting healthy has sold over a million books and helped thousands of people build their best bodies ever, and his work has been featured in many popular outlets including *Esquire*, *Men's Health*, *Elle*, *Women's Health*, *Muscle & Strength*, and more, as well as on FOX and ABC.

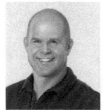

Dr. Cate Shanahan is a health expert who has worked all over the US as a physician and as a health consultant for organizations like the LA Lakers and Primal Blueprint. She is also the author of popular books including *Deep Nutrition* and *The Fatburn Fix*.

Dr. Cate is known for: her 4 Pillars of World Cuisine, explaining why vegetable oils are worse for our bodies than sugar, and her work to eradicate type 2 diabetes through one-on-one consultations. Her work has been featured in many popular outlets including *Men's Health*, *Reader's Digest*, *LA Times*, ESPN, *Sports Illustrated*, and *Good Morning America*.

Dr. Kelly Starrett is a physical therapist and strength and conditioning coach who focuses on strengthening form to minimize injuries and utilizing mobility practices to stay agile. He is also the New York Times bestselling author of *Becoming a Supple Leopard* and co-founder of The Ready State and StandUp Kids along with his wife, Juliet.

Through his mobility exercises and coaching programs, he has helped thousands of individuals, several being top-performing athletes involved in organizations including the NFL, NBA, MLB, UFC, and NHL as well as military personnel and record-breaking Olympic lifters.

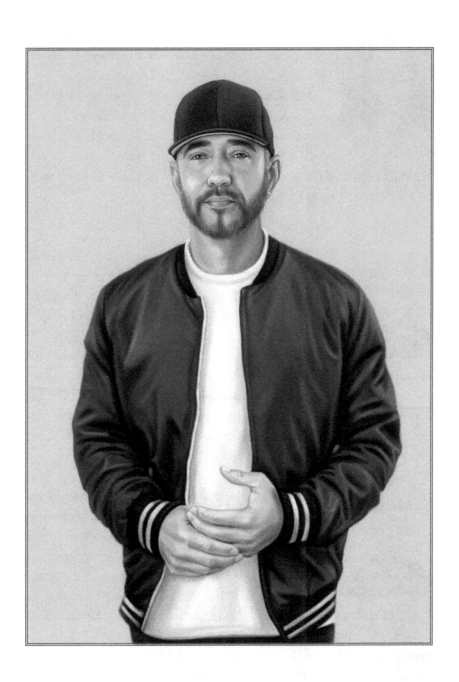

SHAWN STEVENSON

"It's not what you do sometimes, but what you do
consistently, that tells the real story of your results."[1]

Shawn Stevenson is a fitness and nutrition expert who has been working with patients for about twenty years. Whether you are trying to lose weight, build muscle, boost your immune system, you name it, he has extensive content on that topic specifically. Through the platform Shawn built, he has influenced hundreds of thousands of people to improve their overall health and wellness.

It all started when Shawn was in high school. This recollection of his comes from a podcast interview on *Mindcast* with Niels Vium. Shawn was on track to be a star athlete but that came to a quick halt when he broke his hip while running a 200m time trial in practice. He dealt with constant pain and four years later was diagnosed with a degenerative bone disease. When he got this diagnosis, he recalls asking his doctor, "Does this have anything to do with what I am eating?" His doctor looked at him like he was crazy and replied, "This has nothing to do with what you're eating. Just carry on as you are because this is something that just happens. I'm sorry that this happened to you but it's just something you're going to have to deal with. This is incurable."

For the next two years, he followed the doctor's orders of remaining inactive and using medications for his pain. This, along with what he called the "TUF" (Typical University Food) diet, he gained over 40 pounds and wasn't seeing his situation getting any better. Eventually, Shawn said,

"Enough is enough," and decided to take matters into his own hands. He started small: working out on the exercise bike, changing his eating habits, and sleeping better. After six weeks, he lost 20 pounds and within nine months, he reversed the damage done to his bones and amazed his doctors that weren't able to make progress through consultations, medications, and surgeries.[2]

After taking these steps to get his health on track, Shawn kept on improving what he referred to as, "the three pillars of health that changed everything for me: right nutrition, right exercise, and right sleep."[3] He changed his college courses to learn as much on health as he could, got certified as a strength and conditioning coach, and started assisting students and professors at his university with their health and fitness goals.[4] This sparked the start of his career, which has evolved into helping as many people as possible through his books, podcasts, and coaching programs.

On a podcast interview with Mike Dolce (fellow nutrition and fitness expert and UFC weight-cut coach for athletes like Rhonda Rousey and Thiago Alves), Shawn stated that he did not find what he learned in his college courses is what worked with clients. Rather, he felt he had to experiment with a variety of diets including: paleo, keto, vegetarian, and vegan.[5] Shawn goes further into this on another podcast interview for *The Ultimate Health Podcast*, where he explained that he was on a 100% raw food diet for three and a half years. By experimenting with diets, he explains that he learned what works and what holes come with each diet.

A couple other invaluable lessons he took away was:

1. Everyone is unique.
2. It is important to get out of addiction and stop seeking foods like donuts. Instead, listen to what your body really needs.[6]

Shawn took this experience to start a variety projects like podcasts, keynote speeches, and books. After being a podcast host but realizing he was doing the majority of the legwork, he decided to start his own podcast. In 2013, he created *The Model Health Show*, which can still be found at the top of the charts in health and fitness podcasts. Here, he covers all topics and has what he calls "masterclasses" on a variety of topics like Fat Loss, Water, and Blood Pressure. Soon after, Shawn became known as "The Sleep Expert" after releasing his bestselling book, *Sleep Smarter: 21 Essential Strategies to Sleep Your Way to A Better Body, Better Health, and Bigger Success.*

When Shawn is discussing fat loss or health in general, he always has a strong focus on one thing in particular – *hormones.* In *Sleep Smarter,* he states, "Hormones are chemical messengers that deliver information throughout all the cells in your body… We are either supporting normal hormone function or working against it with the decisions we make. We need to eat hormone-healthy foods, practice hormone-healthy exercise, and, as you know, improve the quality of our sleep because it's one of the biggest navigators of our hormones overall."[7]

Two Critical Hormones

The two hormones that Shawn discusses the most in *Sleep Smarter* and *The Model Health Show* are melatonin and cortisol. These hormones strongly influence your sleep – melatonin enables you to down-regulate and prepare for sleep while cortisol enables you to wake up and be alert.[8] When cortisol is low, melatonin is high and vice versa.[9]

Shawn describes melatonin as, "the star of the show when it comes to getting great sleep."[10] It not only benefits your sleep but also your immune system, blood pressure, thyroid function, insulin sensitivity, and more.[11] He describes cortisol as, "incredibly important to the optimal health and performance of your body," and explains that it is crucial for strength, focus, and vitality.[12] Both of these hormones are crucial for regulating your internal clock (also known as your circadian rhythm) which in turn, affects your energy levels over the course of the day. Hormones fluctuate and are regulated by several factors like diet, exercise, and (most of all) sleep.

The Impact of Sleep on Your Health

On an episode of *Muscle For life* with muscle-building expert Michael Matthews, Shawn stated, "Sleep is more impactful on your genetic expression than your diet and your exercise combined and it's because of the huge influence it has on your hormones… and the influence that it has on your immune system."[13] Shawn's awareness of how underrated sleep is in the health space and the overwhelming need for help with his clients' sleep habits is what led him to writing *Sleep Smarter*.

In *Sleep Smarter*, Shawn explains how sleep has a strong influence on your overall health and quality of life as well as how it is affected by so many factors in our lives: stress, nutrition, exercise, etc. He also calls sleep the "force multiplier," enhancing the results we get from our diet and exercise habits.[14]

To show the extents of both the consequences of sleep deprivation as well as the benefits of plenty of high-quality sleep that Shawn calls out in *Sleep Smarter*, here are a couple figures:

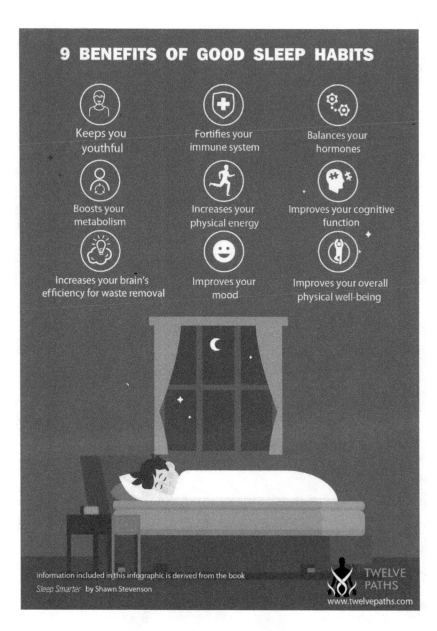

Figure 1: 9 Benefits of Good Sleep Habits[15]

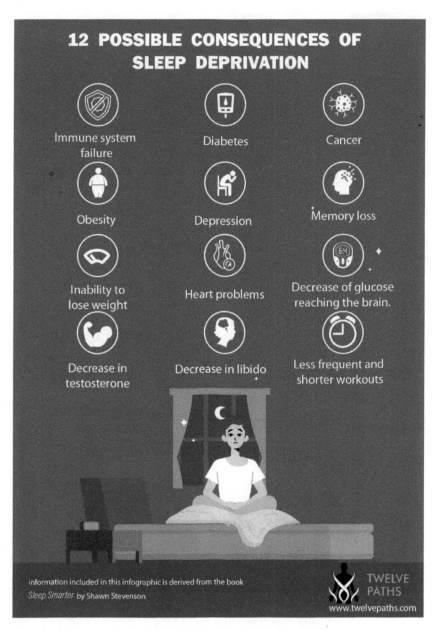

Figure 2: 12 Possible Consequences of Sleep Deprivation[16]

Early Risers Vs. Night Owls

Although the "Possible Consequences of Sleep Deprivation" Figure (**Figure 2**) shows all of the negative aspects, being a night owl isn't all bad. In *Sleep Smarter*, Shawn describes how being a "night owl" or an "early riser" tends to reflect on your character: night owls appear to be more creative, more outgoing, and have a better sense of humor while early risers are better business people, tend to get better grades in school, and are more optimistic, satisfied, and conscientious on average.[17]

This doesn't mean you can't make the change and Shawn does advise being an early riser for the sake of your health. On the same *Muscle For Life* episode that was mentioned earlier, Shawn explains how you can get away with being sleep deprived when you are young but "you're accelerating the point where you *can't* get away with it."[18]

In *Sleep Smarter*, Shawn states, "if you firmly believe you are a night owl and want to make the switch to get your circadian rhythm, hormones, and priorities in order, there are simple steps to do it."[19] To do this, he refers us to Leo Babauta of *ZenHabits.net*'s suggested method of shifting your wake up time by 15 minutes earlier each day until you reach your target time.

To do this, Leo offers the following three tips:

1. Get excited to wake up in the morning. Before you fall asleep at night, think of something that excites you about the morning time. This could be your morning coffee, your morning walk with your dog or significant other, or anything that will make you want to do Tip Number 2…
2. Literally jump out of bed! You'll be much less likely to head back to bed if you're out of bed and enthusiastic about it.
3. Move your alarm clock across the room so that you *have* to get out of bed to shut it off.[20]

Shawn also offers a fourth, bonus tip:

4. "Wake up your senses." Stimulate your senses with something you enjoy when you first wake up. This could be coffee, music, or even just natural light by opening the curtains.[21]

The Benefits of Natural Light

Getting natural sunlight every day is something that Shawn states is crucial to your overall health. In *Sleep Smarter* he states, "Your sleep cycle, or circadian timing system, is heavily impacted by the amount of sunlight you receive during the day... The circadian timing system, along with the scheduled release of hormones, helps to control your digestion, immune system, blood pressure, fat utilization, appetite, and mental energy, among other things."[22]

Shawn explains that sunlight not only regulates melatonin and cortisol production but also actives a neurotransmitter, serotonin. Serotonin strongly affects your mood, bringing feelings of health and happiness as well as increasing your overall quality of life. It is not only affected by sunlight but also by your diet and exercise. To reap these benefits, Shawn suggests getting at least a half hour of direct sunlight each day and states that between 6:00-8:30 a.m. is when you are most responsive.[23]

The Detriments of Artificial Light

Light can also work against you, keeping you up at night and wreaking havoc on your sleep. Shawn states that artificial blue light (from your devices with screens) messes with your circadian rhythm by activating daytime hormones and suppressing melatonin.[24] To counter this, he strongly encourages to make it a point to turn off all screens at least 90 minutes before heading to bed.

Here are a couple other tips Shawn provides to prevent your devices from disrupting your sleep:

- Adjust your settings so you aren't receiving notifications while you're in bed.
- Turn on your phone's setting that switches the blue light on your screen to red light at a certain time. Blue light blocking glasses are also a viable option.[25]

EMFs

As harmful as this blue light can be, Shawn explains that electro-magnetic fields, or EMFs, given off from our devices can be just as (if not even more) harmful. EMFs are given off by all devices (phones, computers, TVs), especially those connected to WiFi.

Just like blue light at night, he says that EMFs disrupt melatonin production, so simply talking on the phone before bed decreases sleep quality and makes it take longer to fall asleep. Shawn also links several other health problems to EMFs, including: leukemia, brain tumors, breast cancer, decreased sperm mobility, and damaged sperm DNA. [26] To avoid these potential problems, Shawn strongly recommends keeping your cell phone out of the bedroom. "It's 99.999 percent likely that you won't miss anything important. But you will radically improve your sleep quality if you're not allowing your cell phone's notifications and radiation to disrupt your valuable sleep."[27]

If you simply cannot do this, he suggests some tips you may find more reasonable:

- Keep any device with a significant amount of electricity at least 6 feet away from you while you sleep.[28]
- Use an electrical timer to turn off your WiFi at night.[29]

A quote from *Sleep* Smarter shows how strongly Shawn feels about this topic – "It's simply that we need to put these things in a more intelligent place in our lives so that we can continue controlling them, instead of having them control us."[30]

There's no question that more people than ever are hooked to their devices before they fall asleep, whether it's their phone, TV, or laptop. In *Sleep Smarter*, Shawn mentions how having a TV in your bedroom has been reported in scientific articles not only to lead to sleep problems but also to obesity and poor grades in children and less sex for adults.[31]

How Sleep Deprivation Leads to Issues with Fat Loss

If you are trying to lose weight, Shawn explains that protecting your sleep should be as important as diet and exercise. To show how sleep deprivation puts us on a path to diabetes, he states, "Studies have shown that just one night of sleep deprivation can make you as insulin resistant as a person with type 2 diabetes."[32]

Shawn covers this topic thoroughly in an episode of *The Model Health Show* titled "The Sleep & Fat Loss Masterclass." In this episode, he describes how fat loss is run by your hormones and your endocrine system and the amount of damage you are doing by only getting 5-6 hours of sleep instead of 8-9 hours each night.

The former (5-6 hours each night) makes you more likely to overeat, increases visceral fat, and negatively affects your melatonin, cortisol, thyroid, human growth hormone (the "youth hormone") and testosterone levels. Some of these are significant changes as well, dropping testosterone to levels as if you were 10-15 years older and increasing your likeliness to choose calorie-dense, carbohydrate filled foods by 33-35%. Meanwhile, if you choose the latter (8-9 hours each night), you can see an increase in fat loss rates by over 50%.[33]

Is 8 the Magic Number?

Many people say that 8 hours is the perfect amount of sleep. Shawn does not agree with this for multiple reasons. Mainly, everyone is a bit different: some people may be fine with 8 but others might need up to 10 hours each night. You also have many lifestyle factors that affect your sleep and certain times are just more valuable than others. According to Shawn, "It's been shown that human beings get the most beneficial hormonal secretions and recovery by sleeping during the hours of 10:00 p.m. to 2:00 a.m. This is what I call *money time*."[34]

There are three stages of the sleep cycle: Non-REM Sleep, Deep Sleep, and REM Sleep, and they repeat (or "cycle") in this order. At the start of the sleep cycle (Non-REM Sleep), your heart rate and your brain activity start to slow down. In the middle of the cycle (Deep Sleep), your body is making repairs and your blood starts to work its way to your muscles. Then in the last stage (REM Sleep), your blood flow in your muscles continues to increase, your heart rate and body temperature increase, and your mind is active so dreams are more intense. Lastly, there is a small interim period of basically being half-awake, then the cycle starts all over again.

Shawn explains that cycles have a typical duration of between 80-100 minutes, so we can predict when we are in each stage. This is helpful to know because having an alarm wake you up while you are in the middle of these cycles can make you feel groggy and exhausted first thing in the morning, whereas if you wake up during the interim period, you should not have that problem since you will be interrupting a lighter stage of sleep.

Here is an excerpt from *Sleep Smarter* where Shawn tells us how to predict this and use this as a tool:

"Sleep cycles typically last for 90 minutes each and repeat four to six times per night. So, six normal 90-minute sleep cycles would equal 9 total hours of sleep... To make your mornings better and more energetic, start setting your alarm so that it goes off in accordance with these sleep cycles instead of the standard "8 hours of sleep." For example, if you go to sleep at 10:00 p.m., set your alarm for 5:30 a.m. (for a total of 7 ½ hours of sleep), and you'll likely find that you feel more refreshed when you wake up than if you set the alarm for 6:00 a.m. and interrupted another sleep cycle."[35]

A couple general suggestions Shawn has to optimize your sleep are:

1. To schedule your sleep around your ideal number of hours.[36]
2. To aim for a bare minimum of four sleep cycles (or about six hours) each night.[37]

Caffeine & Alcohol

Two things that can seriously impair your sleep are caffeine and alcohol. According to Shawn, you should set a caffeine curfew of around 2:00 p.m. the latest[38] and avoid alcohol 3 hours before bedtime.[39]

In *Sleep Smarter*, Shawn explains that caffeine is harmful to your sleep because it causes your body to create adrenaline and cortisol and the half-life is between 5-8 hours. So, if you consume 200mg of caffeine at 2:00 p.m., 100mg could still be active at 10:00 p.m. To explain how detrimental this is, he states that consuming caffeine 6 hours before bed causes a full hour of lost sleep. Some common negative effects are that it brings your base-line adrenaline level down and it can also lead to headaches and migraines when you take a break from using it regularly.[40]

Shawn is not against caffeine and states that, "Caffeine can even be used strategically to enhance metabolism, increase alertness and focus, and even improve liver function if used in the right way... Use caffeine as a boost, not a crutch, and you'll be able to truly enjoy its benefits while still sleeping like a champion."[41]

In an episode of *The Model Health Show*, Shawn reviews a study that showed people who drink 1-2 cups of coffee per day have reduced risk of heart failure, stroke, and coronary heart disease by 8% compared to non-coffee drinkers.

When it comes to alcohol, Shawn explains how it is harmful because of how it disrupts your REM sleep so your body and brain cannot recover properly and your memory suffers as well. He also says that alcohol may affect women's sleep more than men's because they metabolize alcohol faster. Whether you are male or female, alcohol is harmful to your sleep and amplifies sleep issues that you may have currently.[42] One tip that Shawn shares is from a wine expert, Anthony Giglio, who suggests drinking 8 ounces of water with every alcoholic beverage that you have.[43]

One Typical Culprit for Sleep & Health Problems

According to Shawn's chapter in *Sleep Smarter* titled "Get to Bed at the Right Time," there is one thing that seems to trump everything else when it comes to harming your sleep - working the night shift. The night shift has been shown to dramatically increase your likeliness to be sleep deprived which in turn, negatively affects your overall health. Shawn explains how this can increase your chances of getting colorectal cancer, diabetes, cardiovascular disease, and other serious health problems.

Sadly, almost everybody that works the night shift does not have a choice to change things and many of them are the people who serve us: doctors, nurses, police officers, dispatchers, emergency medical technicians, and other emergency personnel. Shawn discusses studies that look specifically at emergency medical personnel and how the night shift increases their risk of metabolic syndrome and can decrease their lifespan by up to 10 years.[44]

To push this point, he states, "If health is your number one priority, then don't work the night shift."[45] Again, sadly most people do not feel that they have a choice. Even so, Shawn does have some advice that could possibly help. If you work 2-3 days per week overnight and then go back to normal, he says that it has been shown to be just as bad as working the night shift full-time. He says, "A better approach could be to have 2 months *off* the normal sleep cycle and 10 months *on* the natural sleep schedule where their bodies are in sync with their natural circadian clocks."[46]

Tips to Help with Insomnia

To wrap up Shawn's outlook and advice on sleep, the following is his advice for those with serious sleep problems. In *Sleep Smarter*, he states that insomnia is sometimes caused by your body being too warm and not being able to cool down so that you can enter deep sleep.[47]

If that is the issue, he has a few suggestions:

- Set the temperature in your room to be between 60-68 degrees Fahrenheit.[48]
- Try taking a warm bath 1 ½ - 2 hours before heading to bed.[49]
- Do not wear tight, restrictive clothing (socks, underwear, nothing).[50]

Shawn also states that exercise can cure insomnia. Specifically, he suggests that if you have a history of sleep problems, you should try superset training. This method of training will not only improve your sleep but is helpful for fat loss as well.

To do this, he says to:

1. Choose two exercises of competing muscle groups (for example, legs and chest)
2. Do 8-10 reps, alternating exercises (for example, 8-10 reps of weighted squats and then 8-10 reps incline press)
3. After completing both exercises, rest until fully recovered (about two minutes).
4. Repeat for a maximum of 30 minutes.[51]

Supplements

It could be said that everything discussed so far are lifestyle factors. Fixing things like light, temperature, time on devices, caffeine and alcohol consumption, and exercise are part of our daily routine that indirectly affect our sleep. There is a reason for this: Shawn does have drug/supplement recommendations but states, "Ideally, you *first* need to address the lifestyle issues that are actually causing the sleep problem. If you jump to taking drugs or supplements, then you'll just be treating a symptom and increase the likelihood that you'll develop a dependency on something that can harm you long term."[52]

If you have exhausted all other options, here are three natural herbs that Shawn says can be helpful sleep supplements:

1. "Chamomile is an excellent tea before bed."[53] Chamomile is a mild sedative so it should help you sleep. Some other positive side effects include: reduced pain, reduced inflammation, treatment for skin conditions, and treatment for heart disease.
2. Kava Kava can also be used to treat sleeplessness and fatigue. Some other positive side effects are: reduced signs and symptoms of anxiety, improved mood, and improved cognitive performance.
3. Valerian is the strongest of these three. It is a moderate sedative so it should be reserved for people with serious difficulties falling asleep.[54]

Some sleep supplements that are not natural are: 5-HTP, GABA, and L-tryptophan. Shawn states that these "can be helpful if intently monitored and used with caution."[55]

Shawn suggests that if you plan to use any of these supplements, you should start low and work your way up unless you are totally confident that you know what you are doing. Your size, gut health, stress, and many other factors affect what amount of a supplement is best for you.[56]

You may even find that these supplements simply don't help. "It's unique to you whether something is going to be helpful or not. This goes for food, supplements, and even exercise. You have to experiment to find out what is the most intelligent, safest, and most effective long-term choice for you."[57]

Exercise

Shawn explains that daily exercise is not an option. "If you're really serious about being the healthiest person you can be, you'll set your personal exercise appointment and sleep time first, then schedule everything else around them."[58] Exercise brings along incredible benefits - not just looking and feeling better but also improving your metabolism, insulin sensitivity, and hormone function. [59]

In *Sleep Smarter*, Shawn references a study that compares people who do activities like swimming, tennis, or running for about 100 minutes per week to people who only exercise for about 15 minutes per week. By measuring their telomere length, the study found that the former group appeared 5-6 years younger than the latter.[60] Even though the study looks more at catabolic (cardio-based) exercise, Shawn states that anabolic (strength-based) exercise, also known as lifting heavy weights, will give you the best hormonal response and allow you to reach your true genetic potential.[61]

"The research shows that you can stay younger, longer if you have more lean muscle on your body."[62] He suggests focusing on compound lifts like those used in powerlifting – the bench press, squat, and deadlift for the best results.[63] In *Sleep Smarter* as well as in multiple podcast interviews, Shawn refutes the popular myth that many women worry about: that weightlifting makes you bulky.

On *The Wellness Mama Podcast* with Katie Wells, Shawn states, "It is very difficult to get bulky when you are lifting weights. You have to eat like it's your full-time job."[64] On *The School of Greatness Podcast* with Lewis Howes, Shawn explains that one benefit of weightlifting is how it helps you produce more human growth hormone (or 'HGH'). HGH helps with recovery, healing, protein synthesis, and the retention of muscle mass. In this podcast interview, Shawn specifically states that deadlifting at 80% of your one-rep-max is one of the best exercises that you can do.[65]

Many people believe running is the best way to burn fat but Shawn states that this is not true because you can burn away your muscle if you run too much. Rather, on an interview with *The Ultimate Health Podcast*, he suggested an exercise plan of lifting heavy 2-3 times per week and walking for 20-30 minutes each day, minimum. As a takeaway for people at the end of the podcast interview, he recommends starting small by just committing to, "Go for a 10-minute walk today. You know, just get out there and do what your genes expect you to do."[66] Another general tip that he has is to get some form of exercise at the start of your morning.[67]

Grounding

One interesting suggestion that Shawn gives related to exercise is to try to do at least 10 minutes of grounding each day. Grounding is being in the outdoors without shoes, ideally on natural soil. He explains that grounding has a wide range of benefits like reducing stress, inflammation, and pain as well as improving sleep quality, tissue repair, and recovery. Shawn also suggests grounding after a long flight to counter the effects of jet lag.[68]

Getting & Keeping Good Gut Bacteria

If you do not take care of yourself while you have jet lag, Shawn explains that this can lead to metabolic disorders because of how jet lag disturbs your gut bacteria. To keep good gut bacteria (which help regulate your immune and digestive systems),[69] he suggests to "Strive to eat organic, locally grown, unprocessed foods for the bulk of your diet."[70]

By eating processed, nutrient-deprived foods, you cause yourself to overeat and also mess with your hormone function.[71] In *Sleep Smarter*, Shawn lays out ten key micronutrients, along with prebiotics and probiotics, and what foods have them. Unsurprisingly, this list contains an extensive variety of natural foods including: nuts, seeds, fish, meat, fruit, eggs, vegetables, and fermented foods.[72]

Magnesium

Out of all the vitamins and minerals, the one that Shawn stresses the importance of the most is magnesium.

He calls this "one mighty mineral" because it provides a number of benefits including:

- Reducing pain
- Calming the nervous system
- Balancing your blood sugar
- Optimizing blood circulation and pressure
- Balancing blood sugar
- Relieving stress and insomnia[73]

In *Sleep Smarter*, he states that, "Estimates show that upwards of 80 percent of the population in the United States is deficient in magnesium."[74] As mentioned before, Shawn believes natural resources are always better than supplements. He also states, "Green leafy veggies, seeds like pumpkin and sesame, and superfoods like spirulina and Brazil nuts can provide very concentrated sources of magnesium for you."[75]

To supplement with magnesium, Shawn suggests that using a topical application on your skin is the most safe and effective form. Specifically, he instructs to apply it in sore areas as well as at the center of your chest and around your neck and shoulders (4-6 sprays per area) at bedtime for the best results. [76] The reason for applying magnesium before bed is that it helps your body rest and digest.[77]

Optimizing Fat Loss

As you can see, the quality of foods and the micronutrients in them are what matter most to Shawn in terms of nutrition. When it comes to adjusting your diet for weight loss, he suggests that calorie restriction is not the way to go. Shawn states that calories restriction doesn't only not work, but it actually works against you. "Research shows that up to 70 percent of the weight you lose through traditional calorie restriction is coming from a loss of your lean muscle tissue."[78] Rather, he suggests eating less carbohydrates and eating a larger proportion of protein and healthy fats to optimize fat loss.[79]

Shawn states how insulin, your body's main fat-storing hormone, reacts to carbohydrates and, "The first thing to understand is that you are either burning fat or storing fat – there is no in between."[80] In an episode of *The Model Health Show* titled "The Heart Masterclass: Blood Pressure, Blood Sugar, & 4 Steps To Perfect Heart Health," Shawn explains how as insulin levels rise, blood pressure does as well and how high blood sugar can damage your blood vessels and your cardiac nerves. The foods that do the most damage are processed and liquid carbohydrates.

He argues that people who claim cholesterol is a causative factor for heart problems are incorrect and that cholesterol is a crucial reparative compound. To back this up, he states that 50% of people who have serious heart conditions do *not* have high cholesterol and that "sugar is the causative factor for cholesterol being out of whack."[81] Due to its high sugar content, Shawn warns not to eat too much fruit when you are trying to lose weight. "If you're going to make a smoothie, then make a green smoothie with a focus on the *green*."[82]

Water

Something that Shawn states is more important than food to our overall health and longevity is water. In his episode titled "Hydration and Water Masterclass" on *The Model Health Show*, he explains how water is crucial for mitochondrial function (which gives you energy from the food you eat), blood flow, and digestion. When we are dehydrated, he also says that this damages our DNA.

In this episode, he calls out the four best sources of water:

1. Spring water
2. Well water
3. Spring or well water bottled in glass
4. Reverse osmosis water or "structured water"

In another episode of *The Model Health Show* titled "The Truth About Your Water Supply & How Water Controls Your Health," he provides a general suggestion of how much water you should drink each day. He says to take your bodyweight in pounds, divide by two, and that number is how many ounces you should drink. So, if you weigh 160 pounds, he suggests 80 ounces of water each day. Some people may need more, some may need less but this should be sufficient for most people, most days.[83] To make it easier to reach this amount, follow his tips of drinking a large glass of water first thing in the morning and keeping a water bottle with you throughout the day. Lastly, he suggests adding natural flavors from things like sea salt, lemon, berries, and/or cucumbers.[84]

Meditation

Meditation is another thing that Shawn suggests doing every day. In *Sleep Smarter* he states, "Meditation is a skill, a tool, and a necessity to help you relax."[85] Even just 5-10 minutes each day can bring benefits like lowered stress, a decrease in inflammation, increased focus, lowered blood pressure, reduced pain, improved sleep, and more. He suggests finding whichever practice works for you and meditating either first thing in the morning or right before getting into bed. [86]

Shawn describes three forms of meditation:

1. Breathing meditation, where you focus on deep inhales and exhales.
2. Guided meditation, where you are following someone's instruction.
3. Movement-based meditation, like Qigong or Tai Chi.

"So, whether it's a breathing meditation, guided meditation, or movement-based meditation like these, take action to uncover a practice that works for you. The benefits are outstanding, and it only takes a few minutes a day." [87]

Relationships

In multiple podcast interviews, Shawn explains how important our relationships are for creating an environment that influences us to live healthier lives. For instance, on an episode of *Health Theory with Tom Bilyeu*, he states, "If you were to ask me… your relationships are the biggest governing force over all of it because that is the most influential thing on the decisions you make with your sleep, the decisions you make with the food that you eat, the decisions you make on whether or not you're exercising or when or how you do it." [88]

Here are some tips Shawn provides to improve our relationships:

- When arguing, take a moment to put yourself in the other person's shoes. "If you're going to be happy and successful in your relationships, you have to get to a place where you want to be in love and happiness more than you want to win." [89]
- Sleeping in the nude with your partner can increase oxytocin. This will combat stress, depression, help regulate blood pressure, and more. [90]

- Rather than focusing on your phone, TV, or computer, focus on each other at night. "The reality of the situation is that communication is the basis for any successful union." [91] This also may lead to the next point...
- In *Sleep Smarter*, he essentially states that the better orgasm you have, the better you will sleep.[92] He also states, "Research shows that during orgasm, both women and men release a cocktail of chemicals, including oxytocin, serotonin, norepinephrine, vasopressin, and the pituitary hormone prolactin."[93]

To show how strongly he believes in this topic, here is another quote from Shawn in the same interview on *Muscle For Life* mentioned earlier - "I believe that your relationships are the #1 most influential things on your health and your success in life. Hands down..."[94]

Conclusion

Shawn works hard to provide you with information on how to improve your overall wellness and your fulfillment in life. In *Sleep Smarter*, he suggests that by educating yourself through books, podcasts, and audiobooks or going to meet-ups and events that bring you closer to your goals, this will help you feel fulfilled and to develop the life you truly want.[95]

In a podcast interview for *Order of Man*, Shawn recommends looking specifically at where you can upgrade things, setting a specific goal, and taking action in that direction on a regular basis. He states, "You're either moving forwards or you're moving backwards... So, even if you move forward just a little bit every day, you're getting closer and closer to making that very specific tangible goal a reality."[96]

By taking this knowledge and making small changes each day to some area in your life, whether you're improving your sleep, nutrition, exercise, relationships, or mindset, you're setting yourself up to be the best version of yourself. At the end of *Sleep Smarter*, Shawn has a "14-Day Sleep Makeover," which guides you on making small changes each day to implement many of the helpful daily habits mentioned throughout the book.

This is the heart of Shawn Stevenson's work: helping people to improve themselves, one step at a time. He continues to work with clients, assist other coaches with their clients through the Advanced Integrative Health Alliance and other programs, speak at events, record podcasts for *The Model Health Show*, write articles, and publish books. At the end of 2020 (the year in which this is being written), Shawn plans to release his new book, *Eat Smarter*. Shawn has been consistently working hard to positively influence others' health over the past two decades and he doesn't appear to be stopping anytime soon.

More Tips from Shawn Stevenson:

- Conventionally-raised cattle are more inflammatory than grass-fed cattle due to higher omega-6 content.[97]
- Many people blame their illnesses on genetics but Shawn states, "Even though our genes play a huge role in our health, they are in no way where the story begins or ends... To put it simply, our environment, our lifestyle, and the decisions we make (either consciously or unconsciously) are determining which genes are getting expressed every second of our lives."[98]
- Light signals your glands and organs (including your brain) to wake up.[99]
- Use your break time at work to get sunlight exposure. Take a walk for 10-15 minutes or at least be near a window.[100]
- "Sunglasses with improper UV protection can be far worse than not wearing sunglasses at all."[101]
- To avoid becoming reliant on caffeine and also avoid building a tolerance to it, take breaks. Specifically, he suggests either going 2 days on and 3 days off or going 2 months on and 1 month off.[102]
- Working the night shift has shown a 30% increase of breast cancer in women.
- Working the night shift also has been shown to double the risk of at-work injuries. "More injuries, more accidents, and a higher rate of mortality are seen consistently for those who are working overnight."[103]
- To keep fresh air in your home, use air ionizers and humidifiers, especially if you can't have the windows open.[104]

- "The sound of running water can actually have an impressive effect on people who have a history of sleep problems."[105] Shawn states that this sound can help slow down your breathing along with your heart rate.
- "Having an intelligently chosen houseplant or two can really do wonders."[106] Some plants he suggests are:

  * English Ivy (air filter)
  * Perennial Snake (air filter)
  * Viney Jasmine (improves sleep quality)[107]

- "If there's light in your bedroom, your body is picking it up and sending messages to your brain and organs that can interfere with your sleep."[108] Even a tiny amount of light can increase body temperature and affect melatonin secretion enough to disturb your sleep.
- "Not getting enough sleep, and not sleeping in darkness, will age you faster and suck away your vitality."[109]
- Having a nightlight as a child has been shown to negatively affect your vision later on in life.[110]
- "The alarm clocks with the white or blue digits are more disruptive than ones with red digits."[111]
- "Getting rid of the light pollution in your bedroom is a huge key to getting the most peaceful and rejuvenating sleep possible." Shawn suggests using blackout curtains to protect your room from outside light and using red light, candle light, or Himalayan salt lamps rather than your usual incandescent lights.[112]
- "Conventional moderate-pace jogging is the mother of all long-duration catabolic exercise."[113]
- Having a consistent exercise regimen radically improves sleep for those with insomnia. Benefits are seen immediately but most benefits come after working out consistently for a couple weeks.[114]
- "Outside of a couple days of strength training (which is essential – and many people love doing this already), add some days of additional activities that you enjoy… Find something you love to do, and do it often."[115]

- "Get an accountability partner. Statistics show that having external accountability drastically increases your rate of follow-through… look for someone who's better (at least a little bit) in the area that you need improvement in, and hopefully you can offer them the same in another area."[116]
- Being overweight can dramatically increase your cortisol levels (by as much as ten times), which is a problem for several reasons, especially the harm it does to your sleep.[117]
- When you are sleep deprived, it is more difficult to resist junk food.[118]
- "Give your body a solid 90 minutes (more is better) before heading off to bed after eating."[119]
- If you need a snack close to bedtime, having a high-fat, low-carb snack (for example, nuts) is best for your blood sugar. Carbohydrates cause a spike in blood sugar, leading to a crash that can wake you up.[120]
- "Have your first meal be an epic one… *Keep insulin down through the first part of your day.* The morning is the ideal time to get in your real food, superfoods, and healthy fat supplements because you're right next to your cabinets at home."[121]
- Alcohol throws off your homeostasis, or your balance of wakefulness and fatigue.[122]
- People with disrupted sleep cycles are more likely to show signs of Alzheimer's disease.[123]
- "'Being awake for 20 hours straight makes the average driver perform as poorly as someone with a blood alcohol level of 0.08 percent, now the legal limit in all states.'"[124]
- "Drowsy drivers are responsible for one in six – or 17 percent – of fatal car accidents."[125]
- One main reason sleep position matters is the integrity of your spine. Your spine will likely be in the best position when you sleep on your back. It also helps with digestion and will help prevent acne and wrinkles. The downside of sleeping on your back is increased odds of sleep apnea and snoring.

- Using too large of a pillow while laying on your back can cause issues with your head, neck, and spine.
- Sleeping on your stomach as an adult can cause issues in your neck and back but can prevent snoring and sleep apnea. Ease tension on your neck and back by lifting a knee, removing the pillow, and/or placing a small pillow beneath your belly and hips.
- Sleeping on your stomach as an infant is critical for development.
- Sleeping on your side appears to be most beneficial for breathing and digestion. If you have a history of back problems, try sleeping with a pillow between your legs while sleeping on your side.
- Sleep-related pain is likely from the sag in your mattress after you've been using it for years.[126]
- Do not reuse mattresses for multiple babies. This has been shown to increase mortality rates up to three times. Also, make sure to use mattress covers for babies and small children.[127]
- "As little as 5 to 10 minutes [of meditation] to start your day will have a cumulative effect on your energy, focus, and ability to sleep smarter. If you ever find yourself in a situation where you wake up too soon and have trouble going back to sleep, simply lie in your bed and practice a breathing meditation to put your brain into the alpha and/or theta state to mimic some of the benefits of the sleep you would normally be missing out on."[128]
- Use guided meditation until you are comfortable enough to get the same benefits without it.[129]
- When using melatonin as a supplement, it is important to know that it is a hormone. "And just like any other hormone therapy... it comes with a greater risk of side effects and potential problems... So, unless you want to chance creating a dependency or shutting down your body's ability to use melatonin, I'd say avoid it or at least try other things first."[130] He later states that it can be used intelligently for short-term instances like adjusting to different time zones.
- "Don't mix sleep aids with alcohol."[131]

- "Go to bed within 30 minutes of the same time each night and wake up at the same time each day… Remember, a consistent sleep schedule is important for your health."[132]
- Massage therapy has been shown to have numerous benefits including: improved sleep increased serotonin levels, decreased pain, stress relief, increased mobility, and more. [133] Shawn suggests using self-massage using tools like foam rollers and/or lacrosse balls nightly and getting yourself a professional massage once per month.[134]
- "This may come as a shock, but a 2009 study found that women who slept in their bras had a 60 percent greater risk for developing breast cancer." This also accelerates the time it takes for breasts to start sagging.[135]
- Wearing tight underwear decreases semen in men.[136]
- Get yourself a small trampoline (also known as a rebounder). Start out with 10 minutes per day and work your way up to 30. NASA has stated that this exercise is the best way to increase bone density.[137]
- Get yourself a Squatty Potty or something equivalent to relieve pressure on your organs while you poop. It is relatively recent that we have switched to sitting instead of squatting to relieve ourselves and Shawn states that this is a very unhealthy practice that cannot only give you constipation, but colon cancer as well.[138]
- Go to the local farmer's market so you can find out where your food comes from and how it's made.[139]
- Working out with your spouse and kids has unbelievable benefits.[140]
- 70% of HGH is produced while you're sleeping.
- The best choice for a probiotic is fermented vegetables.[141]
- "Taking a nap is like a supplement while your sleep at night is the real food." [142]
- Vitamin C is only good as a preventative. It has "little-to-no-effectiveness once you're sick." [143]
- Walking for 20 minutes each day has been shown to reduce risks of dramatic cardiovascular events by 31% and reduce risks of dying by 32%.

- High Intensity Interval Training is good for your heart. Shawn suggests running 20-second sprints (3) with a 2-minute recovery time in between sprints.
- "If there needs to be a change in energy when you walk into a room, bring your best into the room... You are going to influence those around us." [144]
- On a podcast interview with *The Ed Mylett Show*, Shawn references a study that compared calorie restricted dieters that either got 8.5 hours of sleep or 5.5 hours of sleep. The results of this study showed the well-rested group lost 55% more body fat than the sleep-deprived group. [145]
- When you're working, move your phone away from you to prevent what he calls "cyber loafing." Cyber loafing is his term for getting off-task by checking things online.
- "Movement is required for your body to heal." [146]
- If you want to get optimal sleep, you want to get done working out 3 hours before you fall asleep. No closer since this elevates cortisol and core body temperature. [147]
- A study that compared groups of elderly people showed that those who consumed two servings of green leafy vegetables each day had brains that appeared 11 years younger than those who did not. [148]
- On an episode of *The Aubrey Marcus Podcast*, Shawn states how our immune system is greatly affected by our sleep, nutrition, and stress. Just one night of sleep deprivation reduces both production and performance of our natural killer cells. Counter to that, simply going for a short walk can strengthen your immune system dramatically. [149]
- Marijuana becomes a problem when you're addicted to it and can't fall asleep without it. But it can be helpful for short-term use.
- On an interview for *Mind Pump*, Shawn stated that the most common first question he gets from clients is, "What can I take for ____," (improving sleep, more energy, etc.). Shawn's response is, "Always food first, lifestyle first. Supplements can make maybe a 1-5% difference... [Supplements] can be valuable but you have to have the other pieces dialed in." [150]

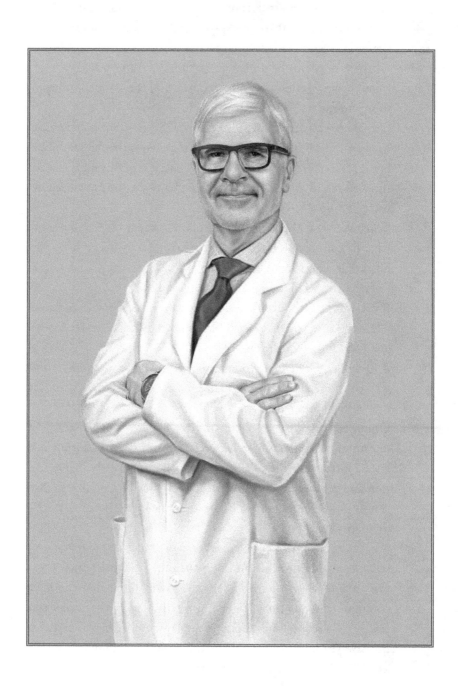

DR. STEVEN GUNDRY

*"I love cardiac surgery. But giving people the tools
to heal themselves transcends just about anything I
can do with a knife, needle, and thread."* [1]

Dr. Steven Gundry has an incredible story of how he made the switch from being a talented heart surgeon to becoming a best-selling author and one of today's well-known nutrition experts. Gundry graduated cum laude at Yale University in the early 1970s and has been heavily involved in medicine (mainly in the fields of cardiology and immunology) ever since. After achieving a medical degree from the Medical College of Georgia, he started on a path to help as many people as humanly possible. Over his career at Loma Linda University Medical Center in California, Gundry and his partner, Leonard Bailey, hold the record for the most infant and pediatric heart surgeries done by anyone around the world.[2] He also holds multiple patents for instruments that other cardiologists use in these surgeries. Dr. Gundry prides himself on keeping patients' hearts alive in a bucket of ice for a long time and the "Gundry Retrograde Cardioplegia Cannula" is one of his patented instruments that does just that.[3]

Big Ed

In the early 2000s, Dr. Gundry had a patient who he calls "Big Ed" that threw a curveball in his career path. Big Ed was a special case who had seen multiple doctors about his clogged arteries and had been continuously told that nothing can be done to help him. After Dr. Gundry had said the same thing, Big Ed explained that he lost forty-five pounds in the past six months and had been taking a number of supplements. Gundry congratulated him on the weight loss and said something along the lines of, "Good for you, but that isn't going to help your heart." Big Ed insisted that a new video be taken of his heart and Dr. Gundry was astounded to find that half of Ed's artery troubles had been wiped away!

On the *Muscle Intelligence Podcast*, hosted by professional bodybuilder Ben Pakulski, Gundry states that prior to this incident with Big Ed, he believed what his education had taught him: that supplements are only good for creating expensive urine. Throughout his career, Dr. Gundry had always been fascinated in research and wrote numerous papers but he had never heard of anything like this. He delved deep into Big Ed's nutrition and realized it had major similarities to his thesis paper at Yale, which hypothesized that apes' diets adapting to the different seasons had caused evolution into the human race.

Thanks to this moment, Dr. Gundry started helping people that he would perform surgeries on to then adjust their diets and start taking supplements so they never had to have the same operation again. He also stated that he had performed multiple surgeries on the same patient several times. In one instance, he operated on someone NINE times. About a year after meeting Big Ed and when Dr. Gundry realized his methods were working, he decided he should be helping people before they ever need surgery so he started his own restorative medicine practice at the International Heart and Lung Institute in Palm Springs, California.[4]

Dr. Gundry's Practice

When he started his practice, Dr. Gundry's patients were mainly overweight men brought in by their wives and he would end up helping both of them because he would soon find the women were almost in just as bad of a condition, if not worse than the men. He still comes across this often today. He states that, on average, the women he helps are on seven different medications when they come to him (usually stomach-acid reducers, NSAIDS like ibuprofen or aspirin, and antidepressants) but believe they are healthy because they eat whole wheat pasta and egg whites.

Dr. Gundry would help his patients by giving them a two-page list of what they were allowed to eat.[5] He takes every chance he gets to thank his patients for trusting in him and being able to run specialized tests (that their healthcare usually took care of) and states that everything he learns is from them. To this day, Dr. Gundry sees patients seven days a week because he loves learning from them and assisting them in bettering their lives by making changes to their diets. His two-page food list is given in his first book, *Dr. Gundry's Diet Evolution*, which was written in 2008.[6]

Using this formula, Dr. Gundry got the nickname "The Fixer" because he had helped many people not only with weight loss but also with several different diseases including:

- Heart disease
- Immune system diseases like lymphomas or multiple myelomas
- Multiple sclerosis
- Lupus
- Ulcerative Colitis
- Crohn's Disease
- Stage 3 Cancers
- Stage 4 Cancers
- Rheumatoid Arthritis

Dr. Gundry's Diet Evolution

Dr. Gundry's first book, *Dr. Gundry's Diet Evolution* published in 2009, appeals mainly to those looking for weight loss tips but overall is a showcase of his root principles along with many of his important dieting lessons. He tells us why so many popular diets (Atkins, South Beach, Orin) don't work because they have so many guidelines and once you break one of them you are off for good and then you gain the weight you lost right back.[7] In Gundry's prescribed diet, there is no counting of any sort - calories, carbohydrates, fats, etc. You simply need to remember the principles and stick to the food list.

This book explains how our genes crave fatty, sweet foods because our ancestors relied on animal fat and sugars from seasonal fruits to survive through the winter. If we follow what our genes are telling us and eat those foods all year-round, we are forcing our bodies to store fat year-round as well. "The internal calorie counter we all carry in our genetic programming activates the killer genes. In other words, death and disease are your genes' way of saying you're being voted off the island."[8] He states how in order to take control of our weight and our lives, we need to fight our genes by staying away from foods that fatten us up like grains and sugars. Gundry goes against what he learned in school. Where they say "a calorie is a calorie," he states "calories merely tell us how much energy is contained in a food, not how much energy your body can derive from it."[9] He goes on to explain how 30% of animal protein is wasted as heat and that carnivores mainly get the nutrients they need by eating herbivores. This is a very important principle showing why he suggests that we ought to eat grass-fed beef, pastured chicken, or wild-caught fish for the little bit of protein we need. He states that most of the nutrition should come right from the source (plants).

Most of the studies Dr. Gundry references, if they are not his own papers or data from his own patients, are studies done on primates. "We share 98 to 99 percent of our DNA with chimpanzees and gorillas. So despite our recent dietary habits… our genes and our fuel needs are most like those of the great apes."[10] One of the most popular quotes in his most recent interviews is that his advice is for us to "live like gorillas who live in Italy."[11] What he means by this is that we need to consume as many leafy vegetables as possible and to drench them in olive oil. Dr. Gundry recommends olive oil as your main source of polyphenols, which help your heart, weight management, and cognitive function. He even goes as far as to state, "the purpose of food is to get olive oil into your mouth,"[12] and suggests aiming to consume a liter per week.[13] Although *Dr. Gundry's Diet Evolution* is a fantastic read with a diet plan that has been proven to work, this book did not give Dr. Gundry the majority of the popularity that he has today.

Dr. Gundry's Transition

In *Big Questions with Cal Fussman*, a podcast where Cal Fussman, one of today's top journalists, interviews highly influential people, Dr. Gundry states how much of a struggle it was to go from being a successful heart surgeon to running his own practice as a dietitian. He states that he and his wife Penny spent all their savings, had their house foreclosed, struggled with car payments, and lived in various apartments for 12-13 years (and he must have been 50-60 years old while this was happening)! Gundry also states how Penny named the day that he looked in the mirror and decided to make the transition from a successful heart surgeon to a dietitian "Black Friday."[14]

On many podcasts, he comically states how dumb it is for a heart surgeon to decide to help people because of how much money they make from doing each surgery. One of Gundry's favorite quotes is from Upton Sinclair, a classic American novelist, who said, "It is difficult to get a man to understand something when their salary depends on not understanding it." This is a profound quote that he uses to explain why he feels many physicians do not have any motivation to learn ways your health can prevent disease - because they are making money off illness.

On the *Diet Starts Tomorrow* podcast, a health and fitness podcast done by two women (Aleen Kuperman and Samantha Fishbein) who talk about the real-life struggles of weight loss and being healthy, Gundry states, "sickness is very good for business... We are in the business of sickness in this country." This is very sobering coming from a man who has helped tens of thousands of patients, young and old. He also talks in this podcast episode of how he was the president of Southern California's chapter of the American Heart Association for two years. He states that the American Heart Association's certified sticker you see on foods in the grocery store is actually purchased. The example he uses is that a grapefruit in Florida will have a heart-healthy sticker but the same grapefruit in Arizona will not because the Florida Grapefruit Association donates $400,000 per year for that sticker. Dr. Gundry also talks about how he has spoken to the American Diabetes Association and how they are working to *maintain* diabetes because they do not believe you can cure or prevent it (*or* because of all the money that comes from the illness).[15]

Even though it was a tough road, Gundry and Penny kept on because he knew he was doing the right thing and his methods were working to help prevent his patients from getting diseases. Regardless of how successful he is now, he says to Cal Fussman that if he knew how rough the transition would be, he probably wouldn't have done it and when Cal asks for advice for an up-and-coming business entrepreneur, Dr. Gundry comically says, "Don't do it."[16]

The Plant Paradox

What has made Dr. Gundry so successful today is his supplement company, Gundry MD (where he is co-owner of a company that includes 600 people), and his first New York Times Bestseller, *The Plant Paradox: The Hidden Dangers in "Healthy" Food that Cause Disease and Weight Gain*, which was released in 2017 and remained as the New York Times Bestseller for more than 30 weeks and continues to be a bestselling book on Amazon.com (#1 in three categories: Vegetarian Diets, Immune Systems, and Paleo Diet).

In Part I of *The Plant Paradox*, Dr. Gundry goes through all of the science and research behind "The Plant Paradox Diet." He states that, "the more fruit I removed from an individual's diet, the healthier he or she became. The more I removed vegetables that have lots of seeds, such as cucumbers and squash, the better my patients felt, the more weight they lost, and the more their cholesterol levels improved!"[17] The book is named "The Plant Paradox" mainly because of how plants can be the answer to good health *or* they can slowly be the death of us.

Lectins are the harmful protein that plants create as a defense mechanism from being eaten, which can be found in things like beans, seeds, and grains. Gundry explains how we all have about 5 pounds and over 10,000 different species of bugs in and around our bodies (making up our microbiome) that either eat good foods like leafy greens and support us to live a longer, healthier life or they eat bad foods (mainly lectins), which take over our minds and make us keep eating bad foods that give us diseases.[18] The "Plant Paradox Diet" is created to cultivate good bugs and eliminate the bad. Dr. Gundry believes this is the answer to managing our weight and immune systems and also preventing disease.

One of the most popular questions Dr. Gundry gets is, "Why is this all of a sudden a problem if we have been eating lectin-filled foods like beans and grains for so long?" He explains how this is a misconception because many of these foods were not discovered until Christopher Columbus "discovered" the Americas, which is not long at all considering how long humans have existed. Our year-round access to so many fruits and vegetables is also very recent; rather than fattening up for winter, we are fattening up year-round on the Standard American Diet.

The fact that we are modifying our foods by using GMOs, antibiotics, and other contemporary innovations is another reason he gives. Rather than our blueberries being naturally small and bitter they have transformed into large sugar bombs.[19] "With the introduction of broad spectrum antibiotics, other drugs, and a vast array of chemicals, we have totally destroyed the gut bacteria that would have normally given us a chance to process these lectins and educate our immune system about them."[20]

Gundry describes how almost all of us are suffering with leaky gut - a condition that takes place when harmful substances (like lectins, for instance) pass through the lining of our gut and into our bloodstream, causing inflammation, fatigue, diarrhea, rashes, allergies, and more.[21] He even claims that leaky gut causes inflammation in the brain that leads to Alzheimer's and dementia.[22]

The Plant Paradox is essentially a handbook on building the mucus along your gut lining so that those harmful substances cannot pass through to other parts of your body or, in other words, building up your immune system. The method he prescribes is to starve the lectin-eating bacteria in your stomach and to slowly work on the number of lectins your body can withstand or to quit eating lectins altogether. Gundry hates the word "diet" and considers this a lifestyle. Most of the foods he allows are green vegetables, fatty oils, nuts, eggs, meat, and fish. The main focus is on vegetables and oils since he believes you should not consume more than around three ounces of animal protein each day.[23]

Similarities & Differences Between Books

"There is evidence that our hunter-gatherer forebears ate about 250 plant species on a rotating basis. Most humans don't even eat a tenth of that number."[24] This is a statement that Dr. Gundry makes in both *Dr. Gundry's Diet Evolution* as well as *The Plant Paradox*. Several common themes show up in both books but there are also some key differences - for instance, *Dr. Gundry's Diet Evolution* focuses on fixing your genes vs. *The Plant Paradox* focuses on removing lectins from your diet and cultivating a good microbiome. One thing that does not change is the fact that all of his science is backed by his thousands of patients that let him take blood markers every three months on things like cholesterol, blood sugar, and triglycerides as he helps them take control of their lives by throwing away prescription drugs and escaping surgeries. Both books are filled with numerous success stories but he also includes several stories where people transition off the diet or start an unhealthy habit like smoking that quickly bring them back to gaining weight or clogging their arteries.

Both books include a similar list of foods to stay away from and a list of foods to keep in your diet (getting rid of grains, most fruit, and almost all processed foods while mainly consuming leafy green vegetables, oils, and certain nuts). Some differences are that back in 2008, Gundry did not have as much of an issue with peanuts or tomatoes as he does today. He gives salsa, tomato paste, and tomatoes in his list of "friendly food" in *Dr. Gundry's Diet Evolution* but in *The Plant Paradox*, with the discovery of lectins, he states you should not consume tomatoes unless you peel and deseed them first.[25-26] Both the "Diet Evolution" and the "Plant Paradox Diet" have structures to them; each consisting of three phases.

Dr. Gundry's Prescribed Diets

Phase 1 is focused on resetting your diet habits. In *Diet Evolution*, he calls this getting out of "store fat for winter" mode and into "winter is now" mode.[27] In *The Plant Paradox*, he gives people the option to skip Phase 1, which includes three days of any amount of green veggies (that are included in his "good" list, of course), certain oils, no more than two servings of avocado each day, and very little pastured chicken or wild caught fish.[28] This phase is meant to restore your gut microbiome, keeping the good bugs happy and repelling the bad.

Phase 2 in both of these books is a repair/restoration phase - where, now that your bad gut bugs/killer genes are warded off, you start truly adapting to the diet. Dr. Gundry asks you to slowly increase your intake of leafy green vegetables while you decrease any calorie-dense foods like animal proteins (which remain on the "good" list, but need to be limited). "The more vegetables you eat, the better your health."[29] He recommends that those with health problems or those who want to ensure a great lifespan and healthspan may want to stay in Phase 2 permanently.[30-31]

Phase 3 can be summed up with a quote from *The Plant Paradox* - "Remember, your goal is longevity with vibrant health, not just limping along for another year on the planet."[32] This is where you take the diet and make it into a lifestyle. Gundry keeps his principles of lowering your animal protein intake as much as possible and consuming more leafy greens but states that it is okay to wean off of the path from time to time. Treat yourself with fruit or legumes or a bit of Indian white basmati rice but use caution. Eating a variety of foods and keeping a diverse microbiome is great, but you don't want to revert back to the Standard American Diet and destroy your gut. If you cut lectins like gluten completely out of your diet and then months later have a large sandwich or a bread bowl as a treat, you're likely to have irritable bowels, massive headaches, or a similar bad reaction.[33-34]

Dr. Gundry also gives you other methods to experiment with in Phase 3 to improve longevity like intermittent fasting and introducing ketones to your diet. Even in *Dr. Gundry's Diet Evolution* (which, he states was first published back in 2008), he proposes intermittent fasting. This shows how forward-thinking he was and how he trusted the science and facts rather than conventional wisdom. "Conventional wisdom holds that skipping meals is bad for you but conventional wisdom has made you ill, fat, and headed for an early grave."[35] He is very blunt with this statement but this is coming from a doctor that has served thousands of patients and has been working hard to help the obesity epidemic in today's society.

To get a good idea of where Dr. Gundry gets his philosophy from, here are a few of the other experts or studies that he references the most between his books and podcast interviews:

Valter Longo's Fasting-Mimicking Diet

Both Steven Gundry and Valter Longo get the bulk of their diet research from a mix of clinical studies and from studying blue zones (the areas of the world with the longest-living people that exist today). From this research, they have found that a high-vegetable and minimal-animal-protein diet is best for longevity. Valter Longo has dedicated this area of his work to proving that intermittent fasting or alternate-day fasting can not only increases your lifespan but reduce risks for and delay cancers, Alzheimer's, Parkinson's, and strokes as well as reverse type I and type II diabetes. Longo has several articles showing the science behind this on his website, valterlongo.com. Such convincing results have come from past animal and clinical (people) trials conducted by him and other longevity experts that Valter is currently conducting several clinical trials.

Dr. Gundry's most popular reference of Valter Longo is his anti-aging study. This study involves mice periodically having food withdrawn for 24 hours and it shows as much of a 30% increase in lifespan expansion compared to the average life. According to Longo's research, fasting also has benefits like stem cell production, metabolic flexibility, and reduced heart rate and insulin levels, just to name a few.[36]

Another study that Gundry talks about is where Longo shows that a five-day fasting-mimicking vegan diet (approximately 900 calories per day) once per month has the same benefits for significant longevity markers as calorie restriction for an entire month. Calorie restriction, in this case, is referred to as removing 30% of your calorie intake from your daily diet.[37-38]

Dr. Gary Fraser's Studies on Seventh-Day Adventists

In *The Plant Paradox* as well as in multiple podcast interviews, Dr. Gundry references a study done by one of his former fellow cardiology professors at Loma Linda University, Dr. Gary Fraser. In this study, Dr. Fraser studied close to 100,000 people (half of which were on some form of vegetarian diet) and compared their diets to show how diet can influence things like heart disease, cardiovascular disease, cancer, Alzheimer's, Parkinson's, influenza, and more. Fraser and his colleagues did this by recording deaths that happened between 2002 and 2007 and the cause of these deaths, then related those to their respective diets.

Essentially, this study showed how all vegetarians were at less risk of death than non-vegetarians. The two groups with the lowest death hazards were pesco-vegetarians (vegetarians who also eat seafood) and vegans. For every 100 non-vegetarian deaths, there were 81 pesco-vegetarian deaths and 85 vegan deaths (these numbers were adjusted to things like age, sex, race, heavy drinkers, etc.). This fits perfectly with Steven Gundry's diet foundation - a heavy vegetable base with minimal animal protein.

Dr. Gundry states how it is difficult to find a "thriving" vegan and how he has yet to find a vegan without a dangerously low omega-3 index. For this reason, he suggests removing lectins and adding supplements like algae oil, which is similar to fish oil but vegan.[39-40]

The Plant Paradox Diet's Effect on Autoimmune Diseases

Possibly Dr. Gundry's most profound research of his own was shown at a presentation for the 2018 EPI Lifestyle Conference hosted by the American Heart Association. In multiple podcasts, he talks about these results and how changing your microbiome can turn genes off and on. He recorded the progress of 102 patients that came to him with symptoms/biomarkers representing autoimmune diseases and/or inflammation and their progress after placing them on the Plant Paradox Diet. Some of the diseases involved were Crohn's, Colitis, rheumatoid arthritis, and lupus. After nine months, 95 out of the 102 had no markers for these diseases. Dr. Gundry used himself in this study, being able to turn on his ApoE4 gene, which is related to Lupus, and then turn it back off through going back on his diet plan. That is not all, the 7 others had reduced markers and 80 out of the 102 now had been taken off of all biologic and/or immunosuppressive drugs. Gundry's focus did not turn to autoimmune disease until after *Dr. Gundry's Diet Evolution*.[41]

Dr. Gundry's Personal Diet

Dr. Gundry would tell you that it is important to find a nutrition plan that works for you, but let's take a look at what his personal nutrition plan is...

- Gain weight with fruit in the winter to lose it in the summer. Eating fruit seasonally, as our ancestors did. As much as he says "give fruit the boot," we all enjoy sweets and getting polyphenols from berries is definitely beneficial. Perhaps doing this increases your metabolic flexibility as well, keeping your gut bugs happy and not starving them out completely.

- Start each morning with a refreshing walk with the dogs. He calls this his form of meditation and a ritual like this is a great one to adopt to relax and set the tone for the day.
- Every year for over a decade, from January through June, he has a two-hour eating window, from 6:00-8:00p.m. This is an extreme exercise of intermittent fasting and does not prescribe something this drastic in his books (in *The Plant Paradox* he prescribes fasting two days a week, for at least sixteen hours each).[42]
- His dinner usually (if not always) consists of him and Penny sharing a massive salad with a wide variety of greens, mushrooms, olive oil, and other nutrient-rich vegetables.
- From seeing how well supplements work with his patients, he is a strong believer and makes sure both him and Penny get their daily dose of supplements like vitamin D, fish oil, and magnesium.

Conclusion

Dr. Gundry trusts the science that tells us our genetics do not control our health and he works to prove this through the work he does to prevent diseases and extend people's lives. His model example and goal is to live like one of his patients, Edith Morrey, who was walking in heels and walking her dog until she passed away peacefully at home at 105 years old, which then led to Dr. Gundry writing his next bestselling book, *The Longevity Paradox*. In *Diet Evolution* and *The Plant Paradox*, Dr. Gundry shows his interest in longevity by helping us achieve "dying young at a ripe old age" through adopting a healthy, sustainable diet that eliminates processed foods and strengthens our guts.

Above all else, Dr. Steven Gundry is a dedicated researcher. With Big Ed, he noticed what he had done was profound and that he had to find out exactly how Big Ed fixed his own heart issues. As a world-renown doctor, he created life-saving devices to keep hearts alive longer during surgery and held records for pig-to-baboon heart transplants. He has written hundreds of articles on all different topics and relies on his own patients as well as other profound experts to keep on learning and help his patients as much as he can.

There are many places to find Dr. Gundry's work:

1. One of his many books - *Dr. Gundry's Diet Evolution, The Plant Paradox, The Plant Paradox Cookbook, The Plant Paradox Quick and Easy,* or *The Longevity Paradox.* If you wonder "what *can* I eat on his diet," a large portion of his books included recipes that are very well-done and worth giving a try. A few great recipes include his Green Smoothie, Dr. G's World-Famous Nut Mix, Paradox Crackers, and Mint Chocolate Chip - Avocado "Ice Cream."

2. On his website, gundrymd.com, Gundry and his team share articles about lectins, longevity, supplements, and hundreds of topics in between. You can learn more about him, find great recipes, or look into the supplements that he sells to keep your good gut bugs happy. You can also sign up for his newsletter through his website which he uses to directly send you links to interesting articles.

3. Dr. Gundry has many podcast interviews since he is such a well-respected and knowledgeable nutrition expert. He also has his own podcast. On *The Doctor Gundry Podcast,* he gives tips on health and longevity, interviews many other experts in related fields, and answers questions that he gets online through Facebook, Instagram, Twitter, or YouTube.

4. All of Dr. Gundry's podcasts are also on YouTube. On his YouTube channel, which is named Dr. Gundry and has almost 150,000 followers, there is a whole world of information including recipes, tips like "The truth about artificial sweeteners," "Alternative types of salads," "Gardening tips from Gundry," you name it.

More tips from Dr. Steven Gundry:

- "The purpose of food is to get olive oil into your mouth." Do your best to consume 1 liter of olive oil per week.[43] By studying blue zones, learning from his patients, and researching studies done by other trusted experts, this is the best thing you can do to live a long, healthy life. Stay away from corn oil, soybean oil, and canola oil. He also says MCT oil is good, especially for those who are ketogenic dieters.[44]

- Pressure cookers are a great thing to have in the kitchen if you can't get away from beans and other lectin-containing foods. Pressure cookers are safe and easy to use and almost completely destroy all lectins other than gluten.[45]

- More than 80% of Dr. Gundry's patients are deficient in Vitamin D3 and "anyone in my practice with leaky gut or an autoimmune disease has low levels." Dr. Gundry states that this essential vitamin prevents leaky gut as well as bone degeneration. He also relates a lack of Vitamin D to prostate cancer and obesity.[46] Take at least 5,000 IUs per day and if you have an autoimmune disease, take 10,000 IUs per day.[47]

- Most people are also deficient in omega-3s and Dr. Gundry prescribes fish oil for this. Omega-3s supply DHA, which has been shown to improve cognitive function, joint health and heart health.[48]

- Artificial sweeteners are no better than regular sugars since any sweet substance tells your brain to produce insulin (which, in turn, tells your body to store fat).[49]

- "Research has shown that it takes at least six weeks of continuous practice to instill a new habit."[50]

- Cinnamon, selenium, and chromium are great supplements that lower blood glucose and insulin levels as well as help with sugar cravings.[51] Gundry also suggests increasing salt to reduce cravings.[52]

- It is great to take probiotics (supplements that supply you with good bugs), but they are not helpful without prebiotics or what he calls "fertilizer" for good bugs. Garlic, onions, mushrooms, and artichokes are good natural sources of the "most beneficial" prebiotics - fructo-oligosacharides.[53]

- "Limiting animal protein - and let me remind you that a fish is an animal as well - extends healthspan and lifespan."[54] This point is emphasized in both *The Plant Paradox* and *Dr. Gundry's Diet Evolution*.

- "My research has shown that if you can work your way up to consuming the equivalent of one bag of dark green leaves (lettuce, spinach, or other greens) daily, your life will change dramatically for the better."[55]

- To increase overall happiness and to better your life - get a dog. Dr. Gundry has actually written prescriptions for dogs and has received feedback from these patients saying that it is the best thing a doctor has ever prescribed. They give you a reason to go outside and they show more unconditional love than any other animal.[56]

Shared thoughts/ideologies:

- "Sleep more, weigh less."[57] This relates to one of Shawn Stevenson's most powerful messages in his book *Sleep Smarter*, where he proves this statement with science on how our circadian rhythm affects our hormone function, the choices we make, and more. Dr. Gundry also provides research that shows direct correlation between not only sleep and weight loss but also between sleep and longevity.[58]

- In Shawn Stevenson's book, *Sleep Smarter*, he says "You are what you eat ate."[59] Dr. Gundry says this as well in his books and in multiple podcast interviews. What they are expressing by saying this is that what animals eat affects their nutritional value. For instance, a grass-fed cow will have a heavier dose of omega-3 fats, while a grain-fed cow will consist of more omega-6 fats. Gundry takes this point further and states how omega-6 fats are related to increases in inflammation and that increasing our omega-3s will decrease inflammation.[60]

- "If you lift weights, you will lose weight."[61] This also relates to one of Shawn Stevenson's key messages. Shawn goes more in-depth than Dr. Gundry by stating that both men and women should be lifting heavy weights regularly and how this is a necessity to be considered "healthy." Gundry believes in certain movements (walking, squats, push-ups, etc.) but also warns you about overstressing your body. He explains how running long distances or overworking your body affects your genes - "strenuous exercise, on the other hand, is rarely pleasurable and sends the opposite message: You are struggling to survive and are not a good example to keep around."[62]
- "Most adults become profoundly deficient in magnesium, a mineral essential for muscle contraction and nerve conduction."[63] Shawn Stevenson does not promote many supplements but this is one that both him and Dr. Gundry recommend strongly. Dr. Gundry also explains how magnesium is given to heart surgery patients intravenously in order to normalize heart rhythm and control blood pressure.

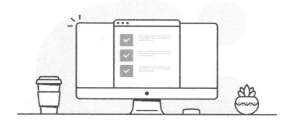

If you enjoy this book, you can also check out my free content at www. TwelvePaths.com or www.InspiringLeadersCollective.com!

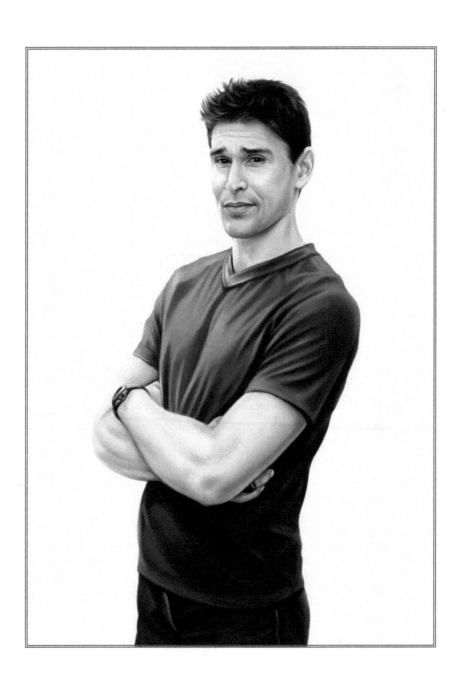

BEN GREENFIELD

"The ultimate goal is to be maximally equipped with the knowledge to build a body that expresses the ideal combination of health, longevity, and performance."[1]

Ben Greenfield is a health and fitness coach for top-performing athletes and fellow CEOs. He is also a competitive spear fisher, bow hunter, and obstacle racer.

Ben has many other roles and accomplishments. Here is a list of just some of them:

- Coach/trainer for endurance athletes and personal trainers
- World renowned speaker on health, fitness, and productivity
- CEO of his supplement company, Kion, which he calls his "playground for supplement formulations"
- Author of over a dozen books
- Ex-bodybuilder
- Blogger/writer as "Get-Fit Guy" for *QuickandDirtyTips.com* and podcaster with *Get-Fit Guy* between 2010 and 2017
- Blogger/writer for his website *BenGreenfieldFitness.com* and podcaster with *Ben Greenfield Fitness* since 2008
- Athlete that has competed in over 100 races and over a dozen triathlons

- Voted America's Top Personal Trainer in 2008 by the National Strength and Conditioning Association[2]
- Named one of the most influential people in health and fitness by *Greatist.com* in both 2013 and 2014 among names like Robb Wolf, Layne Norton, Gary Taubes, and Richard Simmons[3-4]

Ben's interest in performance optimization all started when he was a young, homeschooled teenager in Oklahoma and his parents built a tennis court on their property. Young Ben was attracted to his tennis coach so he started doing what he could to impress her by practicing, educating himself, and training with dumbbells in his room. To this day, Ben plays tennis on a weekly basis. He also has never let go of his love for reading and writing books on both fiction and health/fitness.

Ben finished his high school education at the young age of 15 and then went on to obtain his Bachelor's Degree in Exercise Science and his Master's Degree in Physiology and Biomechanics at the University of Idaho. While he was in college, he planned on going to medical school and was accepted to six different schools but turned down all of the offers. This choice was made after doctors he had worked with told him it would not be smart to become a doctor - an occupation where you can afford to buy a yacht but not have the free time to ever be on it.

Coming out of college, Ben opened his own personal training studios where he used high-speed cameras and collaborated with physicians to evaluate his clients' performance. This is what brought him to be voted America's Top Personal Trainer by the National Strength and Conditioning Association and this lifted him to become the world-renowned speaker, podcaster, and author that he is today.[5]

Ben's main focus is human optimization by ways of improving health and fitness. He not only exercises his due diligence when it comes to research, but shares his extensive knowledge through his books and articles. Whether it's diet, exercise, or lifestyle, Ben also self-experiments with everything that he advocates. He has absolutely no limits when it comes to experiments, including supplements, lasers, enemas, LSD, and stem cell injections.

Essentially, he has experimented with anything that shows any evidence of either health or performance benefits. Ben is known to read around 300 books per year and if you listen to an interview featuring him, you will see how he really is an endless pool of knowledge. His main past experience is with triathlons and assisting athletes at that level. Now, he is an obstacle course athlete and trainer and, as you'll see, even with how much Ben continues to accomplish, he continues to be strong in his purpose to "empower people to live a more adventurous, joyful, and fulfilling life."[6]

Get-Fit Guy's Guide to Achieving Your Ideal Body

Ben's foundation is really built from what he calls "time in the trenches." Between the numerous years of self-experimenting and being a personal trainer/health coach to thousands of people, there is no room to argue that Ben does not know what works. In his book, *Get-Fit Guy's Guide to Achieving Your Ideal Body*, he quizzes you to figure out the body type you have and follows that up with the workout routines he would prescribe in order for you to optimize your body.

More than half of this book is in the "Appendix" section, where he goes into things like: how to measure your body fat, proper gym etiquette, the importance of warming up before a workout and cooling down after a workout, the best methods of stretching, etc. Even if you know the basics, this book is an extensive guide to help you learn about different body types, how to expect your body to change when you exercise based on your body type, and what type of workouts will get you in the best shape possible.

Beyond Training

Apart from being an ex-bodybuilder, world-renowned speaker on health and wellness, coach to a countless number of individuals, blogger, podcaster, and CEO, Ben is also a New York Times Bestselling author with his book *Beyond Training: Mastering Endurance, Health, & Life*. "This book is about how the average athlete can train for endurance while maintaining the delicate balance between health and performance."[7] Ben gives insight on all of the underground tactics of recovery and the science behind things like High Intensity Interval Training and Cold Thermogenesis. He put a full lifetime's worth of knowledge in *Beyond Training* and allows you to "geek out" on several topics in each part of his book. He separates the book into 5 parts: Exercise, Recovery, Nutrition, Lifestyle, and The Brain.

Beyond Training starts out by explaining how there are two different triathletes:

1. Triathletes that eat the Standard American Diet with an overload of carbohydrates and calories while also overtraining consistently.
2. Triathletes that pay attention to what they eat, exercise casually every day with bursts of High Intensity Interval Training, give themselves the recovery their body and brain are asking for, and test their hormone levels, lipid levels, and other measures through blood tests and adjust their lifestyles and supplements accordingly.

Ben then goes deep into of how different these two lifestyles are.[8] 58-year-old Chad (Triathlete #1), suffers from injury after injury, sleep apnea, occasional stomach and digestive issues, dry skin, arthritis, erectile dysfunction, and no time for his family or social events. Ben states, "Chad will ultimately stop getting any enjoyment out of life."[9] On the other hand, 53-year-old Kirsten (Triathlete #2) has just as great of a body but also has a great sex life, nice skin, and, "has never let herself get stuck in a training rut or let her focus on fitness become so time-consuming or all-encompassing that it detracts from her health, her hobbies, her career, her family, or her friends."[10] This book is Ben's guide on how to train like Triathlete #2 - achieving high performance while increasing longevity.

Ben has stated numerous times in interviews that he is featured in that training for triathlons and competitions like them are not something he wants to do for health/longevity reasons, but it is a passion of his to push himself to his limits and he wants to help others do the same while doing the least amount of damage to their bodies.

Becoming a "Fat-Burning Machine"

As far back as seven or eight years ago, you can hear Ben talk to experts like Dom D'Agostino and Peter Attia about their fat-burning/ketosis experiments on the *Ben Greenfield Fitness* podcast. "My own experience with a low-carbohydrate diet began with an attempt to lose extra holiday pounds, followed by the stark realization that, contrary to my expectations and what I had been taught in traditional sports-nutrition classes, my performance, focus, and energy levels actually improved despite a lower carbohydrate intake."[11]

From then on, Ben started putting his clients on similar diets, customized to their own genetics and body types, and was seeing similar results. In his book, *Beyond Training*, and in interviews with other experts, Ben states that since a low-carbohydrate diet helps lower your blood sugar levels, it has several other benefits like reducing risks of endometrial, pancreatic, and colon cancer, cardiovascular disease, cognitive impairments like dementia and Alzheimer's, kidney disease, and diabetes.[12] If you are an athlete, you may like to hear how Ben simply trains his athletes to pay attention to how they look, feel, and perform rather than counting calories and using a scale every day. According to Ben, as long as you eat nutrient-dense foods and take the time to get to know how your body and performance are affected by what you eat, that's what is important when it comes to nutrition.

In 2014, Ben had been on a ketogenic diet in order to be a test subject for a research study conducted by a student attending the University of Connecticut. This study was called the FASTER study (Fat Adapted Substrate use in Trained Elite Runners) and it was a well-monitored and invasive procedure prepared by Dr. Jeff Volek. Dr. Volek is a physician who has developed a clinically proven method of reversing type 2 diabetes by using the ketogenic diet without any medications or surgery.

Essentially, the FASTER study took twenty elite runners (in the top 10% of America's ultra-marathoners) ranging from 21-45 years old, ten of which were on a high-carbohydrate nutrition plan and the other ten were on a low-carbohydrate/ketogenic nutrition plan. What makes this study unique is that all of the low-carbohydrate athletes were on this low-carbohydrate diet for an average of twenty months (ranging from nine months to thirty-six months) so, in theory, they were "fat-adapted," or more capable of burning fat for fuel rather than people on different diets.

On average, during a three-hour long run on a treadmill, the high-carbohydrate group were shown to be burning 0.75 grams of fat per minute, while the low-carbohydrate group were shown to be burning 1.2. This rate even reached over 1.5 grams of fat per minute at times! This is significant because studies before this showed 1 gram per minute being the highest possible fat oxidation rate and Dr. Volek would state that this is because this was the first study where the low-carbohydrate athletes were truly fat-adapted. The study states that 88% of the low-carbohydrate group's fuel was from fat, while only 56% of the high-carbohydrate group's fuel was from fat, on average.[13]

Ben still feels having the ability to burn fat along with carbohydrates is important and he states that he'll usually consume 100-200g of carbohydrates from things like sweet potatoes, wild rice, and greens towards the end of each day. He has tested his ketone levels and finds that by fasting, he can be in ketosis for a good portion of the day even after carbohydrate-loading the night before.[14]

Ben has written several articles that show the benefits of being a low-carbohydrate athlete, stating that you don't need any more than 600 calories from carbohydrates each day, even as a triathlete. In one article, "How I Ate a High Fat Diet, Pooped 8 Pounds, and Then Won a Sprint Triathlon," he ends with, "Folks, these are small changes that will make a huge difference in your life, your health, and your physical performance. I'm not just talking about shedding some extra fat or getting sick less. I'm talking about getting your body to the next level of superhuman performance."

You may be wondering about the "Pooped 8 Pounds," which is in the name because he used a Squatty Potty right before the race and, "had the most liberating, enlightening bathroom experience of his life," so he credited that product for helping him cut some weight right before the race and keep him feeling as clean as a whistle during the race.[15] In almost any article you read or interview you listen to featuring Ben, you'll find he has a very interesting/quirky sense of humor.

In another article, "Rewriting the Fat-Burning Textbook Part 1," Ben highlights the differences between his low-carbohydrate diet recommendations versus what Gatorade Sports Science Institute (GSSI) promotes. Multiple GSSI articles state that athletes on the day before a heavy workout should be consuming at least 3.5 grams of carbohydrates per pound of bodyweight while some go up to even 5.5 grams per pound! If you are 150 pounds, that's 525-825 grams or 2100-3300 calories of carbohydrates compared to the 600 calories that Ben recommends.

GSSI suggests that your carbohydrate fuel comes from pasta, bread, cereal, fruit, and other foods in the same category. During a race, they prescribe sugary gels and drinks. Ben goes on to state, "however, if you desire a long, high-quality life, you don't want to be a washed up ex-exerciser with diabetes, or you don't want to experience joint, nerve and brain inflammation, damage, and degradation, you may need to adjust your lens." From his experience, going from a similar diet to what GSSI prescribes to trying diets like Atkins, Paleo, raw vegan, and the ketogenic as discussed earlier, Ben says, "the #1 prevailing characteristic that defines how good or bad I feel on any of these diets is the amount of sugar and refined carbohydrates, regardless of any parameters (e.g. milk vs. no milk, legumes vs. no legumes, etc.)" He also has given this advice to his clients and reports positive results in both blood biomarkers and performance.[16]

Some other benefits besides performance and feeling good that Ben states a low-carbohydrate diet has are:

- Increasing your body's metabolic efficiency and flexibility (being able to burn both fat and carbohydrates at the appropriate times)[17]
- Improved "appetite satiety and dietary satisfaction"
- Faster recovery[18]
- Reducing your risk or managing certain diseases like type 2 diabetes and cancer[19]
- Ability to maintain lean muscle mass[20]

Although it has several benefits, Ben warns that everyone should be careful in their approach if they do want to switch to being "fat-burning machines." He recommends low-carbohydrate dieters to heavily increase their vegetable consumption in order to increase their fiber and also limit their intake of protein because it can cause their bodies to produce toxic amounts of ammonia.[21] In Ben's article "7 Supplements That Help You Perform Better on a Low Carbohydrate Diet," he recommends several things like extra sodium, amino acids, taurine, MCT oil, glutamine, and magnesium every day. Each of these has their own purpose like improving fat/carbohydrate utilization, boosting your energy levels, or relaxing your muscles.[22] Ben created an entire book, *The Low Carb Athlete*, on this topic specifically.

Mark Sisson is another former high-level athlete that suggests a similar diet to what Ben does. Mark has also written multiple books, runs his own blog, and is CEO of his company *Primal Blueprint*, whose paleo-friendly products can be found in most grocery stores. You can listen to Mark Sisson and Ben Greenfield together on the *Ben Greenfield Fitness* episode "Primal Endurance: How to Escape Chronic Cardio & Carbohydrate Dependency & Become a Fat Burning Beast" or on another *Ben Greenfield Fitness* episode where they talk about Mark's book, *The Keto Reset Diet*.

Biohacking Your Environment

One of Ben's key points of discussion is that we live in an era where we should take advantage of "better living through science." He states that we should always use natural things first, but to use science and technology if it is proven to improve our health and performance. For instance, he suggests to use sunlight when you can, but having an infrared light in the office also works well. Or if you are on a diet with restrictions, he suggests supplements like liver extract, fish oil, or superfood blends but first, try to eat several servings of natural vegetables, fish or grass-fed beef that is high in omega-3 fats, or liver every day.

Ben is considered one of the world's most influential biohackers. In an interview on the podcast *Living 4D With Paul Chek*, Ben shares his own definition of biohacking: the idea of "attempting to increase either the efficiency or the quality of some aspect of human biology using technology."[23] Some solid examples of Ben's "biohacks" involve: controlling circadian rhythm, recovering faster, and reducing exposure to electro-magnetic fields.

Controlling Circadian Rhythm

Ben's current job is mainly being a health and wellness coach for "wealthy, high-achieving, hard-charging executives" and one of the most crucial things they need help with is sleep. He has several hacks for traveling overseas while minimizing the effect on your energy levels and all of them include either light, grounding (contact with the earth), food, or sound. For instance, when Ben is traveling to a different time zone, he will blast himself with light at the times he would normally wake up in the time zone he is traveling to 1-3 days before his flight. He also is a big fan of blue light blocking glasses when it is later in the day to avoid damage to the eyes and to help with circadian rhythm.

Ben uses blue light as a tool to wake up when he needs to, having installed blue incandescent bulbs in his office and gym, and simply avoids it when he's giving his body/brain a rest, so he uses red incandescent bulbs in his bedroom. Ben strongly suggests you switch your phone to remove all blue light at a certain time (most touch screen phones now have this feature) and to install black-out curtains in the bedroom to minimize light exposure as much as possible.[24]

Ben also suggests that you make contact with the ground, preferably with bare feet, as soon as you can after a long flight. This is somewhat anecdotal and follows research done by Joseph Mercola (an osteopathic physician who is also a 3-time New York Times Bestselling Author) but Ben states that "grounding" significantly impacts his sleep in a positive way.

Ben will normally fast while he is on the plane and wait to eat it until it is a normal time in the area he lands in. For example, if he lands somewhere at 4:00 p.m., it may be time to eat dinner back home but he will fast until 7:00 or 8:00 p.m. where he landed and then eat. He also states that if you are somebody who has trouble sleeping, you should not skip breakfast because that is a cue for your body that you are starting the day and it will affect your hormone levels throughout the day and into the night.

When it comes to sound, Ben suggests using soft earbuds while you are sleeping and using a couple apps where you can listen to white noise, brown noise, pink noise, etc. or binaural beats. These can help you fall asleep as well as improve your sleep quality. Binaural beats are music made for "brain-wave entrainment," guiding your brain to work in a certain frequency.

When you are sleeping, these are the brain states related to the frequency of your brain waves:

- Pre-Sleep = Alpha wave brain state (8-12 Hz)
- REM Sleep = Theta wave brain state (3-8 Hz)
- Deep Sleep = Delta wave brain state (0.1-3 Hz)

So, whether you are trying to fall asleep faster, or increase time spent in REM or deep sleep, Ben recommends binaural beats.[25] He also states that bringing your brain into an alpha state during workouts has been shown to be beneficial for performance.[26]

Recovering Faster

Since most of Ben's audience consists of athletes, performance is another popular topic that he covers. The Miami Heat, for instance, hired Ben as a consultant - "it's kinda fun to spend a couple of days down there in America Airlines Arena and visit with their strength conditioning coaches and their staff about how to optimize the players' health and kind of biohack the team a little bit."[27] Never mind the hundreds of triathletes/bodybuilders he has guided through personal training and thousands he has helped through his podcasts, books, and articles. To biohack performance, Ben focuses the most on recovery methods.

"You can't turn your body into a metabolically efficient, fat-burning machine through training alone. Recovery is a big part of the equation."[28] Ben states that there is one major thing people forget to pay attention to when it comes to recovery. The soreness you feel is your musculoskeletal system's need for recovery but you also need to make sure your *neuromuscular system*, or your fight-or-flight nervous system, recovers. You can quantify this with Heart Rate Variability.

"[Heart Rate Variability is] referred to as your HRV or your overall nervous system score. And I know if that's above ninety I really truly am recovered and I'm ready to go smash it. And if it's below ninety and I ignore that, and I pushed through, and I work out hard even though my nervous system is still beat up, I inevitably within a few days, get some kind of like sniffles, or injury, or soft tissue nagging ache and pain, or something showing me that my neuromuscular system wasn't fully recovered. And so it's almost a way to adjust your training on the fly."[29]

Most heart rate monitors with a chest strap can test your HRV and Ben takes five minutes first thing in the morning to test his HRV so he knows what level of a workout he should have that day.

Aside from HRV, Ben states that utilizing heat and cold are the best ways you can take action to recover faster and relieve some of the muscle pain. Due to several health benefits like increased blood flow, Ben does 15-30 minutes of infrared sauna each day. "My daily forays into my infrared sauna are just as important to me as sleep, exercise, and a healthy diet."[30] The infrared sauna is said to penetrate deeper into your body than a dry or wet sauna.

According to Ben's research, the best time to expose your body to this kind of extreme heat is immediately after a workout because it allows you to generate much higher human growth hormone levels. If done appropriately, Ben states that it can have the same effect as doping.

Some of the other benefits Ben talks about in his article, "The Science of Saunas," include:

- Heart health and longevity
- Detoxification
- Immune system boost
- Skin rejuvenation
- Better sleep
- Increased stress resilience[31]

As much as Ben loves his infrared sauna, he advocates cold baths or cold showers even more. In his podcast interview on the *MindBodyGreen Podcast*, he states that cold thermogenesis, or CT, is like "Viagra for the whole body."[32] His thoughts on CT mainly stem from a neurosurgeon, Dr. Jack Kruse.

Dr. Kruse believes that CT allows athletes to reach a level that others can't. He has been featured on *Ben Greenfield Fitness* multiple times and in an episode called "How You Can Use Cold Thermogenesis To Perform Like Lance Armstrong and Michael Phelps," one of Jack's final remarks is, "...knowing what I have in my head now, I wouldn't waste one bit of time dedicating two or three years to become cold-adapted because I think the performance gains are going to astound people."

Dr, Kruse credits Lance Armstrong and Michael Phelps to being among the first high-level athletes to utilize cold thermogenesis but states that they don't publicly share the results because they want to keep their edge over competitors. One of the most fascinating studies that he mentions is one that showed Navy SEALs that are cold-adapted did better at target practice after being dunked in 32-degree water than SEALs that were not cold-adapted. They also did better at target practice than if they were dunked in warm water.

Kruse advises taking 50-55-degree cold baths/showers as much as possible. He also states that swimming is a great way to adapt to the cold, so swimming in a naturally cool river or lake, like Ben often does, may be even better than a bathtub.[33] Ben says that CT improves performance by increasing metabolic efficiency, VO_2 Max, and brain function. In *Beyond Training*, he also states, "Cold thermogenesis can help keep you at a lean racing weight and also improve your cardiovascular efficiency, your immune system strength, your health and longevity, and your metabolic efficiency, thus enhancing your ability to burn more fat during endurance workouts or races."[34] Lastly, in Ben's first podcast with Joe Rogan, he states that testing cold adaptation (being able to sink your whole body into a cold pool or bath with minimal discomfort) is a great way to test your immune system function.[35]

Reducing Exposure to EMFs

Someone who appears to have influenced Ben even more than Dr. Jack Kruse is Dr. Joseph Mercola. Ben admires Dr. Mercola's deep research into scientific studies and their shared desire to learn about things that affect your health and wellness that the average people don't usually think twice about. Electro-magnetic field exposure, or EMF, is one topic they talk a lot about together on *Ben Greenfield Fitness*. In *Beyond Training*, Ben states how the radiation coming from things like your computers and household appliances "can cause headaches, vision problems, anxiety, irritability, depression, nausea, fatigue, disturbed sleep, poor physical performance, and loss of libido."[36]

The biggest culprit that Ben points out seems to be our Wi-Fi. Ben suggests either getting rid of Wi-Fi altogether and using only ethernet cords or at least putting a timer on your Wi-Fi router so you are not getting exposed to the radiation while you are sleeping. He also strongly suggests putting your devices on airplane mode whenever possible because that will drastically reduce the radiation they give off.

In *Ben Greenfield Fitness* episode "How to Reverse the Damage from Cell Phone Radiation, Hidden Sources of EMF, The Best Way to Measure Your EMF Exposure & Much More with Dr. Joseph Mercola," Ben and Dr. Mercola share several hacks you can use to reduce exposure to EMFs. Ben is a strong advocate for all plug-ins being grounded, dirty electricity filters in your home, and grounding pads for under your laptop and under you while you sleep. Dr. Mercola goes as far as suggesting that you have a special sleeping bag that blocks all EMF exposure. A few simple ways to counteract EMF exposure are: to simply avoid using technology, to unplug everything when you visit hotels including the TV and alarm clock, and to utilize grounding.[37]

Parenting

Perhaps the most interesting and profound thing about Ben's way of life is his approach to parenting. Ben and his wife, Jessa, have twin boys at the age of 11 named River and Terran. Ben and Jessa have recently decided to take their boys out of public school and start the "unschooling" approach. The boys were involved in the decision as well and happy to make this change. Unschooling is an approach where the usual curriculum of Math, Science, History, Gym and other subjects still exist but they are aligned to the person's interests and taught mainly by real-life experiences rather than sitting down all day, learning at the same rate as everybody else, and being taught "how to be a good factory worker."

For their Math, River and Terran will be building a tree fort with a tutor who will teach them construction methods using Geometry. This will also teach them a little bit of Architecture. For their Science, they are focusing on health and when Ben teaches at conferences, the boys will be with him, learning.

Cooking will also be a major part of their curriculum. The boys already have their own cooking podcast named *Go Greenfields*, which is their own small business where they make money through advertisements and they also host live cooking shows. Their History curriculum consists of books and movies on topics/time periods that they're interested in learning more about. Lastly, for their Gym, they have a tutor teaching them a Jiu-jitsu class once a week, which Ben joins for, and they also have tutors for other courses like Spanish.

As a family, the Greenfields also have been on multiple wilderness survival retreats and at the age of 13, Ben believes they will be ready for a rite of passage that involves days alone in the wilderness with a coach advising them and checking in on them as they hunt and forage for their own food. They will have times where they are fasting and they will be in solitude, with no devices. At the end of this journey, Ben plans to introduce them to their first "ego-dissolving mechanism," either psilocybin or THC. Ben is well-educated on this topic and states that the dose he plans to give them has been shown not to harm the brain or endocrine system. He believes a rite of passage like this is very important, especially for boys since they do not have a set point in time where they pass into manhood and Ben advises other fathers to do something like this as well. This is definitely a fringe subject and may seem "out there" but Ben is confident in his approach, which he explains in more detail on his interview called "The Ultimate Unschooling Adventure with Ben Greenfield" from the podcast *Front Row Dads*.[38]

Ben's Self-Experimentation

Anyone who knows Ben Greenfield before reading this would be dumbfounded that I've written this much without getting into a few things that he is most well-known for. For instance, if you google "Men'sHealth Ben Greenfield", you'll find several articles he has written for *Men'sHealth*, including a few on penis enhancement. He is not shy about sharing this and the experiments he did for *Men'sHealth*, which included things from gas station pills to soundwave therapy to injecting his penis with stem cells in three different spots.

Ben continues to use his own stem cells, intravenously (not in the penis) every so many years, to inject himself with younger cells and he states that this not only significantly improves his performance in the bedroom but also dramatically improves muscle recovery. Some other things that Ben is well-known for are using coffee enemas (mainly for liver detoxification) and shining an infrared light panel on his testicles each day to soak up the several benefits like anti-aging, recovery, inflammation reduction, etc. As you can see, Ben will experiment with just about anything if he believes it will truly work to help increase performance or longevity.

Conclusion

There are three big reasons why Ben deserves a high level of appreciation for his wealth of knowledge in personal development, whether it be the physical, mental, or spiritual aspect, and his efforts to share this information to positively affect as many lives as he can:

1. His approach of being a student first - learning new information each day from experts around the globe through books, articles, and interviews and digging deep into the science.
2. Ben works hard to serve his purpose and if you listen to his interviews, podcasts, or presentations at conferences, you will see that he forces you to think outside the box to improve yourself. To recall this, "My purpose is to empower people to live a more adventurous, joyful, and fulfilling life."[39]
3. His experience is incomparable and he has always worked to educate not only himself but also those around him.

This may seem like a ton of information but between the number of books and over a decade of articles and podcasts on a wide range of topics, this only scratches the surface of Ben Greenfield. From these resources, you can find specific guides on topics like competing in a triathlon using the most efficient practices, detoxification, replacing the chemicals used in your home with natural substances, increasing testosterone, and what blood markers are most important and what levels they should be at if you are an athlete or are looking to increase your lifespan.

If you look at Ben's career, you can see his progression from focusing on athletic performance to focusing more on longevity. He has always looked for the most efficient ways to be healthy while training for triathlons or whatever your Mount Everest is but lately, he has had a strong focus on longevity, with an effort to blend ancestral wisdom with modern science.

In early 2020, Ben released a new book, *Boundless* which covers an even wider range of topics than *Beyond Training* and talks about optimizing your body, mind, and spirit. Ben stated that this will be his "one stop shop" for everything but since he is always learning more in the realm of health and fitness and experimenting with better living through science, there will surely be more if you choose to follow his work.

More tips from Ben Greenfield:

- Two essentials for living a healthy lifestyle are to have HEPA air filters and reverse osmosis water filters installed in your house to keep your air and water free of contaminants. There are other filters that have the same effect but this is what is in Ben's home and what he suggests. He also recommends adding minerals like sea salt to your water for extra electrolytes and pH benefits (to go even further, if you have trouble falling asleep after a hard workout, he states that 1-2tbsp of sea salt can help get rid of your insomnia).[40]

- The most efficient way of increasing endurance and speed is by "greasing the groove," or doing low-level physical activity throughout the day. Small amounts of push-ups, kettlebell swings, jumping jacks, and other quick high-intensity workouts along with standing and walking as much as possible keeps you healthy while also making you a better athlete. A trick he gives for doing this is creating rules so that whenever you walk under the doorway in your office, you have to do five pull-ups or whenever you enter your office, you need to do five kettlebell swings or kettlebell squats. This has also been shown to increase longevity since you are keeping your body strong without overworking it.[41-42]

- "It seems that fifteen minutes a day of exercise will keep you healthy, thirty minutes a day will keep you fit and lean, and more than ninety minutes a day won't give you any extra benefit."[43]

- Wearing a mouthpiece while exercising (especially during HIIT or resistance training), helps to improve your ability to breathe, prevents the negative effects of clenching, and also lowers cortisol levels.[44]

- "Do strength-training workouts that target the same muscle groups at least forty-eight hours apart... You can, however, do strength training for different muscle groups on consecutive days."[45] In both *Beyond Training* and *Get-Fit Guy's Guide to Achieving Your Ideal Body*, Ben gives workout plans that correlate with this idea by either alternating muscle groups (upper body on day 1, lower body on day 2) or having 3-4 days per week of full-body workouts.[46]
- "Taking 5 to 10 grams of essential amino acids before or during strength-training sessions, and consuming your biggest carbohydrate loads before strength training sessions."[47] Rather than using BCAAs, which only contain three amino acids, he advises that you consume all nine essential amino acids in order to get the most out of each workout.[48]
- "Eat as much protein as your body needs to repair and recover, a little more if you want to put on muscle..." Ben states that in order to maintain weight and give your body what it needs for repair and recovery, you should aim for 0.55 grams of protein per pound of bodyweight. If you are trying to put on muscle, aim for 0.68 grams of protein per pound of bodyweight, there is no need to eat any more than that. Ben states that excess protein can cause dehydration and a build-up of ammonia in your body, which damages your kidneys as well as other organs.[49]
- Add a deload/recovery week every 4-8 weeks of training. Continue to do "injury prevention" workouts, learn new workouts/drills, or do a couple easy fasted workouts. This helps dramatically to reduce stress and is one of the best ways to allow your body to recover.[50]
- Creatine and some forms of DHA like fish oil have a ton of positive research behind them and many more benefits than possible negatives (if taken in normal doses) so these two are good supplements for anyone to take.[51]
- Psychedelics have their benefits in specific roles. For instance, micro-dosing with LSD can increase creativity, psilocybin can dilute your ego, and ketamine can release childhood trauma or help you relive childhood memories. But Ben does not believe heavy doses of psychedelics should be used on a regular basis because of

potential brain issues. He prescribes a wilderness survival technique of being in solitude for days - fasting, meditating, and being in nature as what he calls the "stoic approach" to finding yourself rather than abusing these substances.[52]

- Wearing a mouthpiece during exercise has been shown to increase your breathing capability by over 20%.[53]

- Using CBD oil is another sleep hack that Ben highly recommends because he finds it to be effective to help him sleep wherever, whenever. Typical doses say to use 10-30mg, whereas Ben states to really get the results you want, you need to take around 100mg. He states that this is a good alternative to melatonin because taking melatonin regularly is believed to disturb your body's normal function to create melatonin on its own.[54]

- "According to research, there's a higher calorie-burning response when strength training is preceded by cardio rather than vice versa."[55]

- "When you throw Olympic lifting into your speed-strength mix, the added benefits include increased VO_2 max and decreased resting heart rate."[56]

- Static stretching before a workout can decrease performance and lead to injury. If you are going to hold static stretches, do them after a workout.[57]

- Bone broth, ginger, cold-water fish, and antioxidants are substances that help with mobility, "taking care of your joints and keeping your fascia nice and supple."[58]

- "If your exercise program includes high intensity interval training combined with smart recovery, your red blood cell levels and blood plasma are both going to increase."[59] Doing full sprints for thirty seconds with four-minute breaks in between, repeated 3-8 times can simulate the same effects of running for 5-6 miles and is great for your mitochondria if done a few times per week.[60]

- Start each day with a gratitude journal and involve your family. Ben and his family have used gratitude journals for a long time, and they were always missing something so he created his own *Christian*

Gratitude Journal, where each day you have a quick Bible reading and then you answer the following:

* What am I grateful for today?
* What Biblical truth did I discover in today's reading?
* Who can I pray for and serve today?

- "Whether it's music or art or journaling, having some kind of hobby and engaging in regular learning has consistently been shown to lower stress."[61] Ben strongly advocates playing an instrument for just 20-30 minutes a few times per week.
- "Include a variety of fermented foods in your diet to expose your digestive system to a wide range of friendly bacteria, and your gut flora and immune system will thank you."[62] According to Ben, you should not completely avoid lectins but properly prepare these foods and they should make your microbiome thrive.
- The two key markers to look at for health and longevity, Ben believes, are glycemic variability (how often your blood sugar rises throughout the day) and C-reactive protein (CRP) for inflammation.[63]
- His rule for things that make contact with your skin like sunscreens, dryer sheets, and shampoos is, "if you can't eat it without getting seriously sick, don't put it on your body."[64] This may seem like a crazy concept but we absorb anything that goes on our skin and he states that it does, in turn, affect our health.

Shared thoughts/ideologies:

- In *Beyond Training*, Ben dedicates a whole chapter to sleep which shows that he shares Shawn Stevenson's belief in the importance of sleep. "When I hit this targeted amount of sleep, my workouts are better, my heart rate is awesome, my nerves are sharp, and my creativity and memory are at their peaks."[65] Ben focuses more on jet-lag, apps you can use to track your sleep, and tools like "binaural beats" to enhance your sleep. Ben and Shawn have very similar suggestions when it comes to sleep like keeping devices out of the room, having no light whatsoever in the room, and getting to bed around 10:00p.m. or earlier so that your mind and body can recover as much as possible.

- Ben and Shawn advocate using mini-trampolines or "rebounders" to improve muscle strength and bone density. Ben actually believes vibration platforms give the same benefits but work better.

- Ben and Shawn suggest getting as many nutrients as possible from whole foods. They still believe there are important supplements, one of which is a green superfood blend. It can be tough to eat the whole bag of greens every day, as Dr. Gundry would recommend, so having a teaspoon of a green superfood blend can get you halfway there on its own.

- Ben and Shawn advise that everyone, especially active people, should be taking amino acids. They both prescribe amino acids before, during, AND after your workout. Ben strongly believes in EAAs (essential amino acids), but understands that BCAAs (branched chain amino acids) are more widely used because they are cheaper and they still work well at helping you stay focused during your workout and helping with muscle growth/recovery.

- Ben and Shawn use stevia as a healthy alternative to sugar.

- Ben and Shawn advocate turmeric/curcumin for its anti-inflammatory attributes.

- Ben and Shawn strongly believe that breathing is one of the most important things to work on. Both of them look to breathing for meditation benefits but Ben also describes using correct breathing methods to reduce injury during workouts and controlling your heart rate in extreme situations like deep diving or in ice water.[66-67]

- Ben has a similar diet program as Dr. Steven Gundry, except it is modified for a performance athlete. Essentially, Ben encourages people to eat most of the same foods (olive oil, coconut oil, avocados, wild-caught fish, grass-fed beef) and to avoid most of the same foods (legumes, bread, processed sugars, non-organic meats) along with a heavy focus on vegetables being beneficial. Ben is just less strict on limiting daily calorie and meat intake.

- Like Dr. Gundry, Ben references Valter Longo's fasting-mimicking diet and follows this 5-day diet four times per year. Ben strongly believes in the benefits of fasting for recovery and for our digestion.
- Ben agrees with Gundry that MCT oil and coconut oil are overrated and that if you were to consume one oil in massive amounts, it should be extra virgin olive oil.
- Both Ben and Dr. Gundry warn that too much protein has shown to hurt your longevity. Aim for around 0.55g per pound of body weight and try to consume wild-caught fish or grass-fed beef for the majority of this protein for the sake of obtaining enough omega-3s in your diet.

Contradicting thoughts/ideologies:

- Dr. Steven Gundry and Ben Greenfield believe that Vitamin D_3 is one supplement everyone should be taking. Where they differ is Dr. Gundry states that he has never seen a case of Vitamin D toxicity so he does not see an issue with taking too much. Ben, on the other hand, recommends 35 IU per pound of body weight per day but states that it can be toxic if it is not paired with Vitamins A and K.[68]
- Ben believes that Dr. Gundry's Plant Paradox Diet is too negative about legumes. He states that they are very nutrient-dense foods and they are a popular part of several diets for populations living in blue zones so we should not discount them. If they are properly prepared by soaking or sprouting, they are perfectly fine to be eaten and actually beneficial.[69]

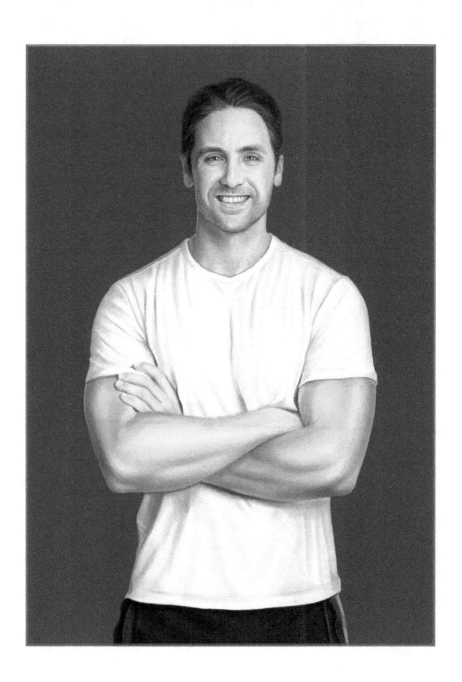

MICHAEL MATTHEWS

"I'm Michael and I believe that every person can achieve the body of their dreams. My mission is to give everyone that opportunity by providing time-proven, evidence-based advice on how to build muscle, lose fat, and get and stay healthy."[1]

Michael Matthews is a health and fitness expert who has helped thousands, if not hundreds of thousands, with obtaining their ideal bodies. Most that have been heavily influenced by Michael have read one of his bestselling books, *Bigger Leaner Stronger,* (or *"BLS,"* his book and program for men), or *Thinner Leaner Stronger* (or *"TLS,"* his book and program for women). His first health and fitness book, *BLS,* was first released in January 2012 and has grown exponentially in popularity ever since. In several interviews, Mike states that he never really wanted to be a "health guru" because he didn't like the people in that space, but he simply wanted to share his knowledge on health and fitness and give a guidebook with the information he wished he had before he started losing fat and building muscle. In *BLS* and *TLS,* Mike gives out his email and personally answers people's questions as a virtual health coach. Since his audience has grown so large and he enjoys helping people so much, Mike has made health and fitness his prime focus.

Mike is now the CEO of a large company, Legion Athletics, that sells a wide variety of supplements, contains a coaching program for reaching your ideal body, and also contains a blog with articles that have been written by him as well as other members of his team that assist him in formulating supplements on their website, LegionAthletics.com. He also started a podcast in 2014 called *Muscle For Life*, where he gives tips backed up by research on a wide variety of areas related to health, fitness, and success. The episodes either include tips that Mike has on specific topics, interviews with experts that have influenced him through their books/programs, answers to the best or most popular questions he gets from his audience through email and social media platforms, or interviews with those who write him with testimonials on how his program has helped improve their lives. Above all, Mike takes most pride in his writing - not only through his blog posts but also his updated versions of *BLS* and *TLS* (which are currently in their third editions) and several other books he has written.

Just about everything in Mike's books is backed up by research he has done, whether from scientific studies published by universities across the globe or meta-analyses done by scientists who have evaluated numerous studies to get a better look at topics like what rep range works best or what micronutrients most people lack.

Mike also has a highly qualified team of researchers that work with him at Legion Athletics to reference. The Director of Research for Legion Athletics is Kurtis Frank, who has an impressive background in supplementation research. Kurtis is the co-founder of Examine.com, a website where you can look up any questions you have on nutrition or specific supplements and get answers backed up by scientific research. His team also consists of several other experienced researchers including doctors and scientists who assist him with supplement formulations and research.

BLS & TLS

In Mike's flagship books, *BLS* and *TLS*, he really shows off his health and fitness knowledge. In the most recent edition of these books, he cites over 500 different resources that are mainly scientific studies that back up his advice on nutrition, exercise, and supplements. Most of his audience is made up of people just beginning their weight loss or muscle-building journey. They either struggled to find anything that works or they wanted to find a guidebook that spells everything out.

Mike states that he was essentially "scratching his own itch" by creating the book that he wished he had access to when he started training. Before he started training, he was 6'-2" and weighed 155lb and now he is up to over 190lb and fit. Mike states that if somebody knows what they are doing with diet and exercise and is willing to put in the work, they can gain at least 20-30lbs of muscle in the first two years of training. Men max out at around 20lbs and women max out at about 10lbs in their first year of training, if they are training naturally (in other words, without the use of steroids).[2]

"Your genetics can't stop you from getting superfit; the knowledge is easy enough to acquire - you're going to learn everything you need to know in this book - and it doesn't require nearly as much willpower as you might think."[3] These books give a complete guide including diet and exercise programs whether you want to gain muscle, lose weight, or just maintain muscle.

One of Mike's favorite ways to give information is by debunking myths that are floating around the health and fitness realm by arguing things like:

1. Why cardio does *not* beat weightlifting when it comes to fat loss
2. How carbohydrates and sugars are *not* what is making us gain weight
3. Why heavy weightlifting is *not* dangerous.
4. Why heavy weightlifting does not make women bulky.

According to Mike, these are all basic things about health and fitness that are important to know. From coaching thousands of men and women, he has learned a ton about what we want our ideal body to be, what body fat percentage and amount of muscle mass is "ideal," and what we need to do in order to get there.

Nutrition

"No matter how many hours you put in at the gym, you won't see major improvements if you're not also managing your diet properly."[4] When it comes to nutrition, Mike states that the "'master key' to your body weight" is energy balance.[5] Essentially, Mike's outlook on nutrition stems from what is called "flexible dieting," which means that as long as you eat the recommended amounts of macronutrients (fats, carbohydrates, and proteins) each day, you will be able to control your physique. "As far as body weight is concerned, how much you eat is *far* more important than what you eat."[6] You will gain weight if you are consuming more energy (calories) than what you burn, you will lose weight if you are consuming less energy than what you burn, and you will maintain weight if you consume the same amount of energy as what you burn.

By going through either *BLS, TLS,* or *LegionAthletics.com,* you can calculate your TDEE (total daily energy expenditure - the number of calories you burn every 24 hours) based on your BMR (basal metabolic rate – the number of calories you burn just to "stay alive for 24 hours") and the amount of activity you get each day. From there, you then calculate your target daily calorie intake based on whether you want to gain, lose, or maintain mass. Here is a figure to show what Mike recommends for both calorie and macronutrient intake based on your goals (which is the same for both men and women):

	Lose Fat (Cutting Phase)	Gain Muscle (Bulking Phase)	Maintain Muscle
Daily Calories	Deficit of 25%	Surplus of 10%	Equal to TDEE
% Protein	40%	25%	30%
% Carbohydrate	40%	55%	45%
% Fat	20%	20%	25%

Figure 1 – Calorie & Macronutrient Guidelines[7-8]

Mike proposes that maintaining weight "shouldn't really come into play until you've completed several cycles of cutting and lean bulking and more or less have the body you want. You use your lean bulking phases to add muscle and your cutting phases to strip away fat, and along the way, assess your physique to see how far you still have to go to look the way you want to look."[9] For men, he also suggests that you should be in the bulking phase until you are around 15% body fat and then cutting until you are back down to 10%, and then repeating. As for women, he suggests bulking until you are around 25% body fat and cutting until you are around 20%, then repeating.[10]

As you can see from **Figure 1**, Mike suggests a high-carb, high-protein, low-fat approach. He states that high-carbohydrate intake is critical for building muscle since your body will mainly be using your glycogen stores (especially with the intense resistance training that his program calls for) for energy and that dietary fat is more easily stored as body fat, which is what you are trying to avoid.[11] Therefore, most of Mike's suggested meals consist of at least 100g of carbohydrates and only around 15g of fat. Even though these macronutrients are important, Mike will argue that you should still practice clean eating and not eat heavily-processed foods like Poptarts for breakfast, lunch, and dinner like other muscle-building experts claim is fine.

Here are some other key things that Mike shares on general nutrition:

- "There is simply no denying that eating too much added sugar can harm our health and that reducing intake is generally a good idea."[12]
- "People who eat more protein lose fat faster, gain more muscle, burn more calories, experience less hunger, have stronger bones, and generally enjoy better moods."[13]
- "You should eat enough [fat] to stay healthy, but have no reason to follow a high-fat diet unless you really enjoy it. And even then, you need to do so with caution."[14]
- "You should get at least 80 percent of your daily calories from nutritious, relatively unprocessed foods. In other words, most of what you eat should consist of whole foods that you clean, cut, and cook yourself, like lean protein, fruits, vegetables, whole grains, legumes, nuts, seeds, and oils. Then, if you feel so inclined, you can fill your remaining calories with your favorite treat."[15]

Another thing to note is that Mike recommends more protein for people who are in the cutting phase than for people in the bulking phase. This is so you can build muscle simultaneously while you are losing fat. He states that as a beginner, this is possible for anybody but once you get years into training, this will really only allow for muscle maintenance since it takes much more effort to gain muscle and you will absolutely need the calorie surplus to do it. For maintaining and bulking, Mike states most people should consume 1 gram of protein per pound of bodyweight per day whereas for cutting, most people should consume 1.1 grams per pound of protein of bodyweight per day (and this is for both men and women).[16-17]

Exercise

When it comes to exercise, Michael Matthews has been serious about building muscle while staying lean for over ten years. After seven years of seriously working out and hitting a major plateau, Mike put down the health magazines and fired his personal trainers and then started teaching himself the proper way to gain muscle and strength by studying scientific research as well as books and programs by some of the best health coaches out there. This dramatically changed his strength and physique and he realized the work he had done in those seven years could have been done in just a few years if he knew what he was doing. Soon enough, friends and family started looking to him for both weight loss and muscle building advice and it was working just as well for them! He wanted to share his knowledge with a much broader audience, so he created his books and programs, *BLS* and *TLS*.

One of the health coaches that he studied, who has definitely had a strong influence on his programs, is Mark Rippetoe. Mark is the most popular interviewee featured on *Muscle For Life* and he also has an extremely popular muscle and strength-building program and book called *Starting Strength*. Mark has been in the fitness industry since the mid-1980s and has taught thousands of people how to properly utilize barbell training through his gym (Wichita Falls Athletic Club in Wichita Falls, Texas) as well as through his international training camps and seminars. Both Mike and Mark's programs revolve around "The Big Three" exercises, the barbell squat, barbell deadlift, and barbell bench press, as the foundation of muscle and strength-building. In *BLS* and *TLS*, Mike goes in great detail on proper form for these three exercises as well as some alternatives. "The stronger you are on these three exercises, the better you're going to look and feel. It's really that simple."[18]

The big difference between Matthews and Rippetoe is that Rippetoe cares far less about aesthetics and more about building as much muscle as humanly possible and maintaining that once you have peaked. In their discussions, Rippetoe states that those that have 8% body fat have psychological problems and will struggle more to gain muscle. On one episode of *Muscle For Life*, Rippetoe states, "I'd much rather deal with an overweight guy than a little skinny guy who's intensely focused on staying underweight and skinny. That guy's got problems..."[19] BLS, TLS, and Starting Strength are all beginner muscle-building programs and teach the principles: energy balance, keeping good form, recovering correctly, etc.

In *BLS* and *TLS*, Michael Matthews explains why he has everyone train mainly with heavy weights, in their 4-6 rep range (80-85% of one-rep max), stopping 1-2 reps before complete failure. His most convincing argument for this is:

> "For instance, a meta-analysis (an in-depth examination of a number of studies) conducted by scientists at Lehman College and Victoria University reviewed 21 studies that compared training with heavier weights (60-plus percent of one-rep max) and lower reps versus lighter weights (less than 60 percent of one-rep max) and higher reps. The scientists found that both styles of training caused similar amounts of muscle growth, but training with heavier weights caused greater increases in strength. One of the researchers, a friend and fellow author named James Krieger, also pointed out... that training with lighter weights only resulted in significant muscle growth when sets were taken to or close to muscle failure (the point where you can no longer keep the weight moving)."[20]

Above all, when it comes to weightlifting, Mike states that progression is most important. Once you reach 6 reps, he recommends that you should immediately add 10lbs to the barbell before starting the next set. If you are a beginner to weightlifting, you should see this progression happening on The Big Three exercises just about every week. As you get further in the program, even if you only progress 1 rep that is something to be happy with.

"*Progressive overload* does [stimulate muscle growth], and more so than any other single training factor. Progressive overload refers to increasing the amount of tension your muscles produce over time, and the most effective way to do this is by progressively increasing the amount of weight that you're lifting."[21] Tracking your progress over time for both your diet and exercise is something that Mike is a strong proponent for, stating that it can make or break your success. He even created an app, *Stacked*, where you can create goals and track your progress with measurements like waist circumference and weight as well as log your workouts.

In Mike's programs, he calls for completing 3 sets of 4 or 5 different workout exercises - starting with the toughest, compound exercises and ending with the easiest, isolation exercises. Compound exercises are those that work multiple muscle groups (like The Big Three) and isolation exercises are those that work a single muscle group (like bicep curls). Mike recommends warming up with your first exercise by doing 2 sets of 10 reps with 50% of the weight you are going to use in your first hard set, followed by 1 set of 4 reps with 70%. For example, if your first hard set is a barbell bench press with a 200lb load, your warm-up includes 2 sets with 100lbs and 1 set with 140lb. Between each warm-up set, he calls for a 1-minute break and another 1-minute break before starting your first hard set.[22]

Here is an example of a workout taken from *BLS*:

1. Warm-up and 3 hard sets with Barbell Bench Press
2. 3 hard sets of Incline Barbell Bench Press
3. 3 hard sets of Dumbbell Bench Press
4. 3 hard sets of Triceps Pushdown[23]

Mike emphasizes doing these exercises exactly in this order, completing all 3 sets for each exercise before moving on to the next.[24] In *BLS* and *TLS*, he also lists other exercises that train the same muscle groups that you can substitute in case you are unable to do a certain exercise (for instance, if you do not have the right equipment). The only major difference between Mike's regimens for men vs. women is that for men, he has more of a focus on the upper body and for women, he has more of a focus on the lower body. This came from his experience dealing with both sexes and what they envision as their ideal body. These programs include 9-15 sets per major muscle group each week.

Some other things he highlights in his program are:

- Using 2-minute rest periods between hard sets when working smaller muscle groups. For larger muscle groups, use 4-minute rest periods.
- Resting major muscle groups for 3-5 days.
- Taking a break from heavy lifting 1-2 days per week.
- Deloading or taking 5-7 days off from training every 8-10 weeks.[25]

Supplements

One refreshing thing about Mike is his outlook on supplements. In his podcast episode, "Making a Good Supplement", he states, "80-90% of results come from your exercise and nutrition. Supplements just speed things up but you can get wherever you want to get to without using them."[26] By having the resources he has and being a CEO of a supplement company, Legion Athletics, that makes eight figures in revenue each year, Mike has a true inside look of what goes on in the supplement industry as well as a very good idea of what works and what does not. In *BLS* and *TLS*, one chapter is called "The Smart Supplement Buyer's Guide" and he takes a deep dive into the six supplements that he believes are most beneficial: protein powder, fish oil, vitamin D, multivitamins, fat burners, and muscle builders.

"I feel comfortable saying that a proper fat loss supplementation routine can increase fat loss by about 30 to 50 percent with few if any side effects."[27] Mike is a strong advocate for using caffeine for both fat-burning and muscle-building because it increases performance, fat loss, and strength. In the same *Muscle For Life* episode mentioned earlier, "Making a Good Supplement," he talks about how caffeine is portrayed as much more dangerous than it actually is. He states that if your daily intake is below 400mg, there are no serious risks for the average active person. Since you build a tolerance to caffeine, Mike suggests to play it smart and "'reset' your tolerance and preserve its effectiveness"[28] by either only using caffeine before your heaviest workouts or, if you are using it daily, to take a week off every 2-3 weeks.[29]

For muscle building specifically, Mike suggests using certain supplements pre-workout and post-workout. The product of his that sells the most is his pre-workout supplement, Pulse. For those that want a cheaper alternative, he suggests that you purchase caffeine pills, citrulline malate, and beta alanine.[30] His post-workout prescription consists of mainly using creatine and protein powder. Creatine is another supplement that people claim is dangerous but Mike argues that, with creatine being possibly the most researched muscle building supplement there is, all evidence shows that creatine is only dangerous for people who have certain kidney problems. Creatine is known to enhance muscle growth, strength, endurance, as well as recovery. He suggests taking it post-workout because it has been shown to be more beneficial than pre-workout and also because caffeine has been shown to downregulate creatine's effects.[31-32]

Overall, the protein powder that Mike recommends for post-workout is a whey protein from a supplier that you trust because it is quickly digested and, "whey is rich in the amino acid leucine, which plays a vital role in stimulating protein synthesis."[33] Before bed, he recommends a casein protein powder due to the fact that it digests slowly so amino acids are steadily released little by little over time. Mike also gives great detail on soy protein, pea protein, collagen protein, rice protein, and hemp protein but these are either more expensive and just as effective, less effective, or lack research compared to whey or casein protein. When it comes to fish oil, vitamin D, and multivitamins, Mike recommends these to everyone to lower their risk for diseases or to improve overall health since our Western diet lacks certain nutrients like EPA, DHA, magnesium, zinc, and vitamin K.[34]

Success & Motivation

Mike's most recent fitness book, *The Little Black Book of Workout Motivation*, goes way beyond the title. In this book, he gives an outline on what it takes to be successful and how to get there. And this success is in anything, not just fitness. Being a father of two and the CEO of an eight-figure company after only being in the fitness industry for a few years, he definitely knows what it takes to be successful. Throughout the book, just like all of his other written work, it is loaded with research. It not only references several scientific articles but also many of his favorite books on success and business and success stories from fans of his who reached out to him because Mike truly helped change their lives for the better.

The Little Black Book gives advice on setting your goals and how to avoid failure at all costs. There are inspirational quotes scattered throughout the book for you to look back to when you find yourself in a slump.

Here are some examples:

- "There may always be another level - but striving to reach the top is the most rewarding adventure life has to offer."[35]
- "No matter what you're facing in life, you have two choices: you can put in the work or get put in your place."[36]
- "The willingness to sacrifice immediate gratification for future rewards is highly correlated with the ability to create a better life."[37]
- "The hard part is taking the stars out of our eyes and considering how much pain we're willing to endure to get these things."[38]
- "You have to give yourself wholly to something to achieve anything worth having."[39]
- "There's nothing that can't be overcome with enough perseverance."[40]

One of the key parts of this book is Mike telling you the first step - to quit doing unproductive things like spending time on social media or watching TV and to focus that time and energy on something that pushes you further in life: whether that be in your career, relationships, or in the gym. As he put it, "I don't care. I'm training. You're not. End of story. So, seriously. Shut up. Shut. Up. And train."[41]

Mike takes this further by stating how many people that reach out to him start by training, but soon enough, end up improving their lives in several other areas. He relates the struggle and dedication in the gym to what it takes to be successful in anything. You won't get anywhere without putting in the work and, if it is something really worth having, suffering.

"The people who win make the right sacrifices and the people who lose don't."[42] In podcasts and books, Mike uses the analogy of life being like cooking a meal, where you only have so many "burners", or things you can focus on, and the more burners you try to use, the more likely something will go wrong. In other words, you need to focus on the few key things that matter most and keep everything else out of your mind. Each chapter of *The Little Black Book* has a "Do It Now" section, where he has you do exercises that either help you find what truly motivates you or give you more discipline. One of the longest but most important exercises that Mike has you do is Warren Buffet's "2 List Strategy," which is used to find your top five goals in the categories of health, work, love, family, and friends.

You start by listing your top twenty-five goals related to those categories. Then, you narrow it down to your top five goals and completely forget about the other twenty.[43] In the "cooking a meal" analogy, you are using 5 burners and focusing solely on these goals and nothing else. *Everything* you do should be pushing you further to one of these goals in order to get where you want to be. Mike gives tips like being as specific as possible and also helps make sure your goals are powerful motivators yet feasible.

Mike has several strong motives for doing the work that he does. His fitness books are not only to help people find a fitness and nutrition program that is simple and works, but in *The Little Black Book* especially, he presses his outlook on how, in today's society, we are too hooked on things that give us immediate gratification (social media, TV, video games) and that none of those things truly give you happiness. Here is a powerful quote from Mike in an episode of *Muscle For Life* when he interviewed another fitness professional, Ru Anderson:

"I think happiness is an outgrowth of pursuing goals that matter to you, that have meaning to you, making progress…where you are spending time doing things that are challenging to you, that you're getting immediate feedback on…you can see your progress, that you lose yourself in… you just don't get that experience from watching YouTube videos all day."[44]

When it comes to Legion Athletics, Mike's major motive is to set new standards for the supplement industry. He raises the bar by publicly revealing tests done on the supplements he sells to show that they do indeed contain what is on the label, in the amounts shown. He also shares the scientific studies that show how these amounts are the clinically effective doses and that the ingredients themselves are effective and related to what the product is supposed to do. In several podcasts, Mike does not shy away from stating what other companies get away with - using fillers like flour, not having the ingredients or amounts of ingredients listed, offering "bullshit products" like testosterone boosters, or adding ingredients in small doses that are ineffective just to be able to advertise the ingredient on the label.

Conclusion

Above all, Mike states that the thing that gives him the most motivation to keep working in the fitness industry is the testimonials that he gets from those who have used his *BLS/TLS* and/or his online coaching programs through Legion Athletics. These personal accounts remind him that he is making a strong impact in peoples' lives, and, often times, not only making them look good but giving them a more fulfilling life overall. When people ask him in interviews what he considers his title, he simply states that he is an author. There are several things to admire about Mike's work: his authentic attitude, the amount of hard work and research that he does for every book, article, and podcast, his willingness to help those who reach out to him, and his dedication to improving the supplement industry as well as the fitness industry as a whole. He works to remind us that muscle-building and "clean eating" are not as complicated as other experts say it is.

Mike's other books related to fitness include *Cardio Sucks*, *The Shredded Chef* (a cookbook to go along with his *BLS/TLS* programs), *The One-Year Challenge For Men* and *For Women* (a year's worth of workouts to go along with *BLS/TLS* laid out to track your progress), *Beyond Bigger Leaner Stronger* (a program for intermediate/advanced weightlifters after following *BLS/TLS* for 2-3 years and hitting a plateau), and *Fitness Science Explained: A Practical Guide to Using Science to Optimize Your Health, Fitness and Lifestyle*.

In the background, Mike and his Legion Athletics team are also currently funding multiple research studies: a lean bulking study looking at the difference of a 5% versus a 15% calorie surplus and a lean gains study involving intermittent fasting.[45] Even though Mike repeatedly states that the fitness industry is "not his scene" and that his real passion is writing fiction books, from the sounds of it, Mike definitely has more to come before he leaves the fitness space.

More tips from Michael Matthews:

- "The best dietary protocol is the one you can stick to, and that's very true in the case of meal frequency."[46] As long as your daily calorie intake is in line with your goals, there is no difference if you have two meals a day or six. One caveat to this is if you have four or five different times in the day where you have a decent amount of protein, that is more beneficial for muscle-building than two or three times, even if you are getting the same amount at the end of the day.

- "Compound exercises produce larger increases in both testosterone and muscle growth than isolation exercises."[47]
- People with larger ankles and wrists have more potential for muscle growth than those with smaller ones.[48]
- To lower your risk for heart disease, limit your saturated fat and processed meat intake (besides red meat).[49]
- "Research shows that athletes who eat low-carb diets recover slower from their workouts and gain less muscle and strength than those who eat more carbs...eating a low-carb diet will reduce your strength and muscle endurance."[50]
- "Anything we can do to reduce stress in our lives and improve mood improves our self-control."[51] In *BLS* and *TLS*, Mike gives some strategies on reducing stress like:
  * Using essential oils like lavender and chamomile.[52]
  * Having sex more often can improve your mood, overall well-being, and your relationship.[53]
  * Get 7-8 hours of sleep each night and limit your blue light exposure before bedtime.[54]
  * Drink green tea.[55]
  * "Studies show that five minutes of low-intensity exercise outdoors is enough to improve your mental state."[56]
- Do your most difficult daily tasks at the start of the day.[57]
- Mike has two 10-minute rules:
  * "Put a mandatory 10-minute wait time in place before you allow yourself to act on a craving or other impulsive urge to do something you know you shouldn't."[58]
  * "If you're dreading something you know you need to do, commit to doing it for 10 minutes and then decide whether to continue. Chances are, you'll find that once you're in motion, you'll want to keep going."[58]

- "We can all benefit from improving our ability to connect our present actions with their future consequences."[59] A couple things that can assist you in this are completing Jordan Peterson's Self Authoring Program (www.selfauthoring.com) or by writing a letter to "Future You."
- Aim to eat 1-2 servings of fruit and 2-3 servings (cups) of fibrous vegetables each day. [60]
- "If you haven't eaten protein in the three to four hours preceding your workout, then it's a good idea to eat 30 to 40 grams before you train."[61]
- Having protein post-workout has been shown to prompt muscle protein synthesis more than any other time.[62]
- Create meal plans in order to keep track of your calories and macronutrients. Also:
  * Use a scale to correctly portion your food.
  * Use websites like CalorieKing when you need to.
- "Occasionally allowing yourself to loosen up can make your diet as a whole more enjoyable and improve dietary compliance and long-term results."[63]
- Pay attention to your physical exertion during HIIT workouts. As you progress, your endurance improves, and you must increase the time you are at a high level of physical exertion in order to continually improve cardiovascular endurance.[64]
- To maximize fat loss, do 1-2 hours of HIIT per week.[65]
- Train your back muscles as much as your shoulders and chest. Also, don't forget to train your hamstrings.[66-67]
- When deadlifting, either wear socks or shoes with flat, hard soles. Also, protect your knees from deadlifting with shin guards, knee-high socks, or knee sleeves.[68]
- "Studies show that inadequate EPA and DHA intake can increase the risk of a number of health conditions, including heart disease, Alzheimer's, and cancer."[69] EPA and DHA are found in fatty acids like fish oil.
- "Insufficient Vitamin D levels is associated with an increased risk of many types of disease, including osteoporosis, heart disease, stroke,

some cancers, type I diabetes, multiple sclerosis, tuberculosis, and even the flu."[70]

- Don't drink your calories unless you are aware of your calorie intake.[71]
- "Start with a baseline water intake of about 0.75 to 1 gallon per day, and add 1 to 1.5 liters per hour of exercise, plus a bit more for additional sweating."[72] 1 gal = 128oz, 1 liter = about 34oz.
- "For physically active people, 2 to 4 grams [combined intake of EPA and DHA] is a sensible recommendation."[73]
- "600 to 1,000 IU of vitamin D per day is adequate for ages 1 to 18, and 1,500 to 2,000 IU per day is adequate for ages 19 and up."[73]
- "The size of your waist is a reliable indicator of fat loss or gain…"[74] Mike recommends tracking weight and waist circumference at the start of each week that you are on his program. For recording weight, he suggests stepping on a scale every morning after using the bathroom and before having any meals and then taking your average for that week since weight can fluctuate.[75]
- "Your hormone health is truly in your hands… Studies show that there are plenty of ways to naturally improve your hormone profile, including staying lean, doing regular resistance training, and maintaining good sleep hygiene."[76]
- Writing down when and where workouts will occur dramatically increases follow-through.[77]
- Don't share your goals with others until you have objective results. This reduces fear of failure and prevents you for giving yourself false satisfaction.[78]
- "Recruit someone you love and trust to hold you accountable to your goals."[79]
- "There's a point where making money might make you feel better about yourself in the abstract, but won't do much for your daily mood… This number is $75,000 per year, but this one-size-fits-all prescription fails to take into account objective factors like cost of living, number of dependents, and inflation, as well as subjective ones like goals and purposes."[80]

- "This is the 'secret' to guilt-free dieting and exercising. So long as you can stick to the plan fairly well most of the time and keep calm when you stumble… You'll never struggle to improve your body composition."[81]
- Relationships have a strong impact on your health and happiness.[82]

Shared thoughts/ideologies:

- Mike and Ben Greenfield recommend the use of reverse osmosis filters for your water.[83]
- Mike and Ben recommend using HIIT cardio rather than long distance cardio. The same study is referenced by the two of them, showing how four 30-second sprints with four minutes of rest in-between is more beneficial than doing sixty minutes of walking with a heavy incline.[84-85] Mike suggests using biking and rowing rather than sprinting if your goal is maintaining muscle and strength while also improving cardiovascular health.[86]
- Both Mike and Ben highlight the importance of deloading/taking days off to allow your muscles to recover and continue to progress. "What I've found is while guys and gals in their 20s can go anywhere from 12 to 15 weeks or longer before needing additional recovery time, people in their 40s and 50s need it more frequently, sometimes as often as every 4 to 6 weeks."[87]
- Mike, Ben, and Steven Gundry all highlight the importance of getting omega-3s in your diet to improve both cognitive and physical performance and suggest supplementing with fish oil.[88]
- Mike, Ben, and Shawn Stevenson all state how sleep is critical for performance and results in the gym. One addition that Mike makes to this is that being in a calorie deficit heightens the negative effects like stunted muscle growth or even muscle loss that you get from not getting enough sleep.[89] All three of these experts also suggest limiting blue light exposure before bedtime since this suppresses melatonin production.

- Both Mike and Ben recommend using heart rate variability to test your overall stress levels.
- "Remember that your health and fitness routines should enhance your life, not consume them!"[90] This is a quote from Mike but this is also a big point that Ben Greenfield makes in his book, *Beyond Training*, where he explains how to train for ultramarathons and triathlons without sacrificing your life outside the gym.
- Both Mike and Shawn recommend limiting your intake of caffeine but also state that it can be useful.

Contradicting thoughts/ideologies:

- Michael Matthews states that there are no studies linking high protein intake to bad health. This goes against how Ben Greenfield and Steven Gundry state that high protein intake negatively affects longevity.[91]
- "BCAAs are worthless and EAAs are even more worthless unless you're into fasting but even then…"[92] This statement goes against Shawn Stevenson and Ben Greenfield's thoughts on amino acids. Mike's thoughts on this are backed by the experts that he works with for Legion Athletics. He states in *BLS* and *TLS* that BCAAs may be beneficial if you are training for several hours per day, "but for the rest of us, it's far more sizzle than steak."[93]
- Mike would argue with Dr. Gundry on the fact that grains make you fat and unhealthy. Mike states that the only real problem with highly-processed carbs like pasta and bread is that they are easy to overeat so he advises limiting these foods if you are not an active person and/or not keeping track of your calories.[94]
- Mike states that CBD is a complete scam because many of these products don't provide the benefits they claim and experts making claims are doing so for financial reasons. This goes against what Ben claims CBD can do.

- In *The Little Black Book*, Mike states, "the entire idea of 'detoxing' the body through cleanses, teas, and supplements is outright quackery..." Ben would argue that there are benefits that he has gotten from doing detoxes periodically and has talked to experts about how these things can be measured. One thing they can agree on is what follows, "... a regular "digital detox" through tech-free time can be well worth it."[95]
- Ben is much more on the hazardous side of caffeine, stating in *Beyond Training* that it can stunt muscle growth, overwork your central nervous system, and lead to adrenal fatigue.
- Shawn argues that calorie restricted diets and limiting fats does not work, whereas Mike states, "if all we're talking about is body weight, then a calorie is very much a calorie, and "clean" calories count just as much as 'dirty' ones."[96]

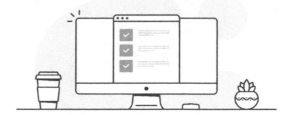

It would mean the world to me if you could take a minute and leave a review on Amazon.com, B&N, or wherever you bought this book!

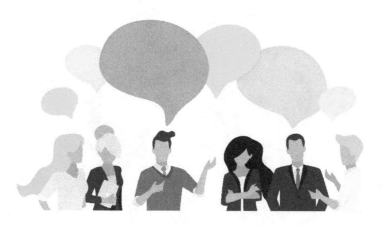

If you're enjoying this book, tell a friend about it! Word of mouth is the best way to make something known.

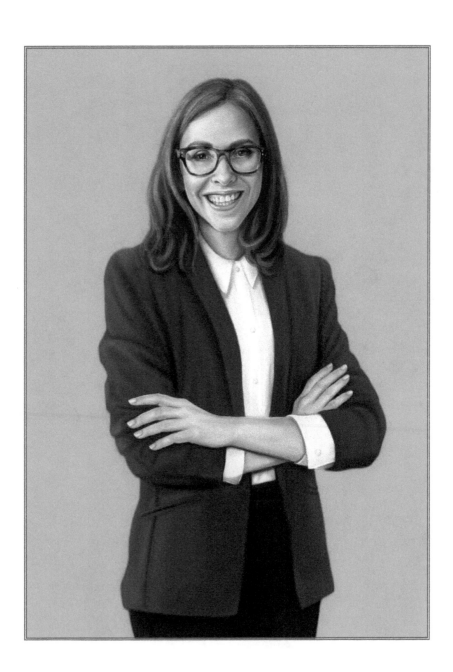

DR. CATE SHANAHAN

"Small steps, repeated often, can lead to massive
health improvements over time."[1]

Dr. Cate Shanahan has been a board-certified family physician for over twenty years. For schooling, she studied Biology at Rutgers University, Biochemistry and Molecular Biology at Cornell University, Medicine at Robert Wood Johnson Medical School, and Family Practice Residency at The University of Arizona. From there, she worked at various medical centers all over the United States including: Washington, Minnesota, Hawaii, New Hampshire, California, Colorado, and Connecticut.

Back in her high school days, Dr. Cate was a top-level runner who got a four-year scholarship and an invite to the Olympic Trials. But soon after that, she started suffering from things like pulled muscles and shin splints. In college, Dr. Cate's goal was to discover why she was having these issues and to help other athletes with similar problems through genetic engineering. When she realized that she will not see anything like this in her lifetime, she changed directions to studying Family Medicine and Nutrition.

Realizing the Power of Nutrition

Between 2000 and 2010, she worked as a physician at the West Kauai Clinic in Hawaii. In a podcast interview on *Get Over Yourself* with Brad Kearns, Dr. Cate talks about how during her time in Hawaii, she noticed that it was common for the grandparents to be healthier than the younger generations, even their grandkids. She took this as proof that our western diet is ruining the health of children.[2]

At this time, she was also experiencing her own serious health problem where her knees hurt so bad that she had trouble walking. She stated that she had talked to five physicians and had surgery but she could not find a cause or a remedy.[3] Not knowing the cause or the cure of her health challenges coupled with her husband Luke's encouragement, she had the inspiration to start something new. Since Luke makes his living through writing, she started working with him on writing her flagship book, *Deep Nutrition*.

The LA Lakers

In 2010, Dr. Cate decided that she needed to move from Hawaii back to the Mainland in order to be able to influence more people. A year or two after moving back, Luke convinced her to send a copy of *Deep Nutrition* to Gary Vitti, the Head Athletic Trainer for the Los Angeles Lakers. He stated that she would be able to assist them with a nutrition plan that would make the players less susceptible to injuries and allow them to recover faster.

Luke was right and Gary Vitti made Dr. Cate a part of the Lakers' training staff, working closely with Gary, Tim DiFrancesco (the team's strength and conditioning coach), and Sandra Padilla (the team's dedicated chef) behind the scenes by creating the PRO (Performance, Recovery, Orthogenesis) Nutrition Program. For over six years, she worked with Sandra to give the Lakers' players as many meals as possible filled with whole, fresh, and nutritious elements.

In an interview with *NBA.com*, Dr. Cate stated, "The most important idea I try to instill in the players is that we need to get away from the idea of food as fuel... Food is the way our bodies communicate most directly with nature... Thinking of food simply as an energy source ignores the other important functions of good nutrition, and that's a fundamental conceptual error that can get folks in real trouble."[4] Dr. Cate's contract with the Lakers made it so she was not able to directly assist any other sports teams but, soon enough, other teams caught on and started using similar practices.

ABC Fine Wine & Spirits

In 2018, Dr. Cate decided to leave the Lakers and move from Newtown, CT to start consulting with ABC Fine Wine & Spirits in Orlando, FL, where she continues to work today. ABC is a company with over 1500 employees and Dr. Cate was hired because the company cares about the health of their employees and would rather have them consult with her to learn the power of changing their diet rather than going through the normal health care system.

In an interview with Richard Jacobs on *Future Tech Podcast*, Dr. Cate explains her work with ABC. She stated that she shares educational resources with the entire company but her main role is to eliminate diabetes using group programs and one-on-one consultations. At the time of this interview, she had worked closely with 120 individuals who began with blood sugar levels in the high 100s or even in the 200s and were taking insulin shots along with other diabetes medications. Two weeks after consulting with Dr. Cate, if they followed her advice, she had gotten them off all their medications, lowered their blood glucose levels by 100, and they also usually lost 20-30 pounds in the process.

Here are the most common tips she gives to people she consults with at ABC:

- Avoid vegetable oils
- Limit how many times a day you snack
- Avoid foods high in calories but low in nutrition (potatoes and rice)
- Avoid foods high in sugar but low in nutrition (fruit)[5]

Public Enemy #1 and its Roots

Whenever Dr. Cate is a podcast guest, she makes sure to call out what she calls "Public Enemy Number One" when it comes to nutrition - vegetable oil. She states that organizations have gotten it wrong when they say saturated fats are the enemy. Polyunsaturated fatty acids (or "PUFAs"), mainly those that come from vegetable oils, are chemically imbalanced and turn toxic from processing methods. In turn, when we ingest these PUFAs, they cause oxidative stress, damaging cells throughout our bodies from our brain to our heart and then to our skin.

On an interview for *The Ready State Podcast* with Kelly and Juliet Starrett, Dr. Cate states that, "the origin of all evil in the nutrition world is the idea that fat clogs arteries." She blames this on a physiologist and professor from the University of Minnesota named Ancel Keys.[6] In the documentary series, *The Real Skinny on Fat*, Dr. Cate as well as other health experts tell the story of Ancel Keys and how he caused the decline in health over the past couple generations and how he has raised rates of almost all chronic diseases.

In the 1950s, the American president Dwight D Eisenhower had a heart attack. In the early 1900s, heart disease was rare and by the 50s, it was on the rise so people were searching for the cause. Ancel Keys took advantage of this and the American Heart Association (or 'AHA') took in his idea that saturated fat and cholesterol clog arteries, which then leads to heart problems.

Being friends with Paul Dudley White, a founding member and president of the AHA at the time, Keys got an enormous amount of funding to conduct his research to prove this. Dr. Cate and the other experts state that there were several flaws with his research including: cherry-picking the regions of the world he studied so that they would back up his hypothesis and blatantly ignoring the fact that the increase in cigarette smoking was also a factor in the regions that he researched.

Dr. Cate states that these studies conducted by Keys led to Procter & Gamble (the manufacturer of Crisco, the first fat used for cooking made out of 100% vegetable oil) funding over 1.5 million dollars to the AHA, which was "the beginning of a very dangerous connection between Big Food Industry and medicine."

Time Magazine also featured Keys in 1961 as Man of the Year and in his interview, this is where he created the image of fats causing cholesterol to clog arteries. Dr. Cate explains that this is wrong because it is not saturated fats clogging the arteries but unstable polyunsaturated fatty acids causing arteries to become corroded and also causing a reaction with iron that forms blood clots. In her interview in *The Real Skinny on Fat*, Dr. Cate ends with a powerful quote:

"So, before we started this experiment, the rates of type 2 diabetes were almost non-existent. But the rates of obesity and our unhealthy diets have so dramatically accelerated that now children at age 2 are being diagnosed with type 2 diabetes and at age 3 and 4 are having complications from it like strokes and heart attacks. So this one idea that saturated fat was bad that came from Ancel Keys was like setting off an atom bomb in our health and it has changed the course of history for human health."[7]

Rather than listening to Ancel Keys, Dr. Cate suggests that we should listen to the science coming from lipid scientists and biochemists.[8] In *Deep Nutrition*, she delves deep into the science of how vegetable oils can cause things like:

- Blood vessels not functioning properly
- Stress on the heart
- Erectile dysfunction
- A lethargic mindset[9]
- Disfigurement[10]
- Alzheimer's
- Learning disorders
- Depression[11]
- Inflammation-related gastrointestinal disorders[12]
- Migraines[13]

To identify the oils you should stay away from, Dr. Cate calls out the 3 C's and 3 S's: corn, cottonseed, canola, soy, sunflower, and safflower. She also mentions that you should stay away from grape seed, rice bran, and refined palm oil. Oils packaged as generic "vegetable oil" are usually one or a combination of these oils. Dr. Cate warns that even if a restaurant or product says they have an "olive oil blend," it is likely a small percentage (as little as 1%) olive oil mixed with other, harmful vegetable oils like canola.[14] Some fats that she suggests are good for you are olive oil, butter, and peanut oil.[15]

Public Enemy #2

Public Enemy Number 2 is something that almost all health experts agree needs to be limited in order to stay healthy - sugar. Dr. Cate states that the main reason sugar is bad for us (and most experts don't explain this right) is that sugar sticks to our cells, which damages them so they cannot function properly.

She shows how this addicting substance leads to:

- Diabetes by elevating blood sugar to irregularly high levels
- Nervous system disorders like recurring infections, joint problems, anxiety, allergic disorders like hives, and more
- Headaches
- Impaired cognitive function, especially in developing children
- Weakened joints, bones, and muscles
- Alzheimer's[16]

"I am not anti-carb. I'm pro-healthy carbohydrate proportioning." That being said, Dr. Cate identifies all carbohydrates as sugar, since both simple and complex sugars (carbohydrates) get broken down into glucose in our bodies. Therefore, for diabetic patients or anyone trying to lose weight, she suggests limiting carbohydrates to 100g per day, whether they come from pasta, rice, chips, cereal, or bread.[17] She suggests that the only time you may need more than 100g of carbohydrate per day is if you are an athlete who does intense exercise like sprinting or heavy lifting.[18] Dr. Cate makes it an important point to state that she is a fan of *all* real foods. The more we process foods, the more we take away their nutrition and natural flavor.

The Relationship Between Medicine & Big Food

A resounding theme throughout *Deep Nutrition* is how big food industries and the medical industry have worked together over the last century to destroy our health. By appealing to peoples' wallets, foods have been engineered to be as plentiful and cheap as possible, with no regard to all of the decrease in nutrition because of it.[19] Dr. Cate relates the foods we eat today, loaded with preservatives and factory-made chicken-flavored seasonings, to pet food and space foods.

By the medical system *treating* illness rather than getting to the root of it, the power of nutrition gets overlooked. The medical system has become a business where the quality (and outcome) of a study comes from the source of funding, where we are being misinformed by studies that tell us sugars are the best/only fuel source and that children should be eating sugar-loaded foods like cereals as soon as they can. "[The medical] industry has moved past selling sickness and learned how to create it."[20]

What Nutrition Courses are Missing

Dr. Cate also shares her disgust for today's education system in the medical industry in several podcast interviews. On an interview for *Real Food Reel*, she states that schools all over the world should be using Weston A. Price's discoveries as the foundation of Nutrition courses. Weston Price was a dentist who traveled the world in the 1930s and discovered how traditional cultures used food to connect them to nature in order to obtain superior genetics. While today, most people fall short of nutrient requirements, Price explained, "the diet of these primitive groups... have all provided a nutrition containing at least four times these minimum [mineral] requirements."[21]

Deep Nutrition

To think back to healthier times, Dr. Cate suggests we do not have to go back as far as the Paleo community makes us think. In *Deep Nutrition,* she provides a number of facts and statistics to show this. For example, she states that the likeliness of women getting breast cancer in the 1960s was one in twenty-two, whereas now it is one in eight.[22] In an interview for The Model Health Show, Shawn Stevenson called *Deep Nutrition* the *To Kill a Mockingbird* or the *Moby Dick* of nutrition books.[23] Most of Dr. Cate's research for this book came from either Biochemistry textbooks, cookbooks from at least a century ago, and TV shows like Anthony Bourdain's *No Reservations* which displayed cooking habits of indigenous cultures.

From observing various different cultures, she realized there were four components that made up all healthy diets, which she calls the Four Pillars of World Cuisine:

1. Meat on the bone
2. Organ meats
3. Fermented and sprouted foods
4. Fresh foods

Meat on the Bone

"Meat on the bone" means that when we consume meat, we should be including everything that comes along with it. Most of the meat you find in the grocery store is stripped of the skin, fat, cartilage, and bones even though all of those things give us nutrients that our bodies need. Dr. Cate warns that the more you cook meat, the less nutrients remain, especially when it comes to steak - she advises trying to work your way down to eating steak medium-rare or even rare.[24] She also states that the bones can be used to create something she calls "a missing food group," bone stock.[25]

Among the many benefits, Dr. Cate highlights the importance of bone stock increasing the health of your collagen. Collagen is the most prevalent protein in our body, making up a large portion of our skin, joints, arteries, and bones. In *Deep Nutrition*, she has a chapter dedicated mostly to collagen called "Forever Young," stating how healthy collagen is great for everyone, whether you are young, old, or a professional athlete because of its capability to prevent injuries and keep you looking and feeling younger.

On a podcast interview for *Fat-Burning Man* with Abel James, Dr. Cate talked about a time where she used bone stock to benefit the Los Angeles Lakers. During a game in the 2013 season, Kobe Bryant hurt his ankle on a play and was estimated to be unable to play for 4-6 weeks. The night of the injury, Dr. Cate made sure to have bone stock sent to Kobe Bryant's hotel room and he ended up only being off of the basketball court for 12 days.[26] She also states how elastin, a type of collagen, is a great measuring tool for life expectancy. "If any single molecule could represent the fountain of youth, this [elastin] would be it."[27] Dr. Cate believes the more the merrier when it comes to bone stock. There are only benefits to having a couple tablespoons of a reduced demi-glace sauce or a couple cups of store-bought broth each day.

Organ Meats

Organ meats are food that Dr. Cate says used to be a very common part of our diet, even here in America, until very recently. She warns that you need to make sure you trust the source but says that liver is, "nutritionally the most outstanding meat which can be purchased." By eating organ meats regularly, Dr. Cate states that children can reach their true genetic potential and adults can do better at resisting diseases.[28] Her general recommendation is to eat organ meats between 1-3 times per week.[29]

Fermented & Sprouted Foods

Fermented and sprouted foods are beneficial because of the microorganisms that are integrated into them. Any seed can be sprouted and some examples of fermented foods are yogurt, kimchi, cheese, sauerkraut, and kombucha. It is important to prepare these foods correctly to avoid molds but, when done correctly, there are substantial benefits to including these foods in your diet.

Dr. Cate states that these microorganisms make foods more nutritious, can provide all the vitamins needed other than vitamin D, and also help prevent several allergic, auto-immune, and inflammatory diseases.[30] Essentially, these beneficial microorganisms, known as probiotics, help us keep a healthy gut and immune system and she recommends having a probiotic-rich food once a day.[31]

Fresh Foods

When Dr. Cate talks about "fresh foods," she is talking about all natural foods: meat, dairy, vegetables, fruits, and seafood.

The keys to this Pillar are:

1. All foods are more nutrient-dense when they are fresh (unless they can be fermented).
2. Fresh foods give your body plenty of antioxidants.

"Remember, cooking burns up antioxidants and damages many vitamins. So the more you eat cooked foods, the more you need to balance your diet by eating fresh, uncooked, pungent-tasting herbs and vegetables."[32] She suggests implementing a rule of fours: having a salad with four cups of vegetables of four different colors, four days a week.[33]

Dr. Cate is a huge supporter of raw milk and drinks it every day in her morning coffee. In *Deep Nutrition*, she argues that raw milk has many more benefits than pasteurized milk including: improved mood, disease resistance, and neural development. She also states that the processing methods used for pasteurizing milk cause the nutrients to be less bioavailable along with a decrease in protein content and an increase in intestinal distress.[34]

The Importance of Nutrition to Pregnancy

One topic that Dr. Cate takes seriously, addressing it both in podcasts as well as in-depth in *Deep Nutrition*, is health during pregnancy. She states that over 70% of women are deficient in nutrients and "if most mothers-to-be aren't even taking in enough nutrients for themselves, how can we expect them to properly provide for a growing baby, not to mention one right after the other?"[35]

Here are some direct examples that Dr. Cate provides, showing which risks are related to which nutrient deficiencies (the following examples are deficiencies that most women have, even *after* taking a prenatal vitamin):

- Vitamin A deficiencies heighten risk for eye, skeletal, and organ defects
- Vitamin D deficiencies heighten risk for schizophrenia, diabetes, and skeletal disease

- Choline and long chain fatty acid deficiencies heighten risk for learning deficits/decreased intelligence[36]

Other nutrient deficiencies and unhealthy diets filled with sugar and vegetable oils also commonly cause negative effects to a baby's body symmetry, height, immune system, vision, and life expectancy along with a lifetime of obesity.[37,38]

Here are a couple important tips that Dr. Cate gives related to this topic:

- Taking a prenatal vitamin *before* conception is most beneficial since the first ten weeks of pregnancy is the most pivotal time for forming the baby.[39]
- "...You should give yourself at least three, probably four, years between pregnancies and make every effort to fortify your body with vitamin-rich foods (or if you can't, at least use prenatal vitamins) *before* conception."[40]
- Low cholesterol numbers lead to premature births as well as smaller babies with smaller brains.[41]

Evaluating a Lipid Panel

When Dr. Cate looks at a patient's lipid panel, she has a much different way of evaluating cholesterol levels than most doctors. She states that an LDL of 70 and an LDL of 150 have a very similar risk of heart attack (15% versus 20%, respectively) while risks for things like cancer, depression, infections, and hemorrhagic strokes go up substantially when your LDL is as low as 70.[42] More of Dr. Cate's thoughts on cholesterol will be discussed later.

Here is a diagram showing how she evaluates lipid panels:

FIGURE 1: Lipid Panel Evalution [43,44]

HDL	LDL	Triglycerides	Triglycerides/HDL	
> 45 in me > 50 in women	< 3 x HDL	< 150		If all correct, "a person's fat-distribution system lipo-proteins, and diet are healthy."
	> 190			Look into family history (possible familial hyperlipidemia)
			> 24	Your body is not handling the fat in your blood well and probably in the process of promoting arterial disease

Other Ways to Test Endothelial Function

Although an endothelial function test can be a good test to show the health of your arteries, Dr. Cate provides a couple alternatives that are cheaper and simpler. The first is fasting blood sugar, which she believes is an underrated measure for general health and diabetes risk. If you have a fasting blood sugar of 89 or higher, she says that this may be a sign that you have predia-betes, which should be taken seriously since it raises your risk for everything diabetes does including: kidney failure, strokes, heart attacks, etc. When she has patients with a higher fasting blood sugar than 89, she recommends they restrict themselves to eating no more than 100g of carbohydrates per day.[45]

The second option for testing arterial health is blood pressure, which is tested at each physical and can also be tested at most pharmacies. Normal blood pressures, to Dr. Cate's standards, are in the ranges of 80-120 systolic and 50-75 diastolic. Getting a reading of 130/80 while relaxed can be a sign of abnormal endothelial function.[46] The reason so many people have high blood pressure and bad health overall is the fact that 66% of the average American diet consists of three ingredients - sugar, flour, and vegetable oil.[47]

If we replaced these ingredients with real, traditional foods, she believes we can reverse the damage the past century has done.

Supplements

As you can see, Dr. Cate is a big proponent for real foods. Normally, she doesn't even like to suggest supplementation of any kind. On a podcast interview with *The Melissa Ambrosini Show*, she states that there are six key minerals: iron, selenium, magnesium, zinc, copper, and manganese and that most of these are accessible with a well-balanced diet. That being said, she states that magnesium and zinc are tougher to come by nowadays and should be supplemented.[48]

For those with dietary restrictions or that do not have access to certain foods, here is a list of supplements that Dr. Cate recommends for you:

- If you do not eat red meat or liver, supplement with desiccated liver pills.
- If you do not eat dairy, bone-in fish, or bone stock, supplement with calcium citrate.
- If you do not consume grass-fed dairy fat, supplement with Vitamin K2 and Omega-3.
- If you are vegetarian, supplement with Iron.
- If you are vegan, non-dairy, or vegetarian, supplement with iodine.[49]

The Fatburn Fix

Dr. Cate's most recent book is *The Fatburn Fix*, which was released in March 2020. While the information she shares in this book is similar to *Deep Nutrition*, this book is not only to inform you but to help you form healthier habits by providing a set of rules along with a program to follow. Dr. Cate states that most diets hurt your ability to use fat for fuel and also damage your metabolism.[50] "[Rather than focusing on weight loss,] you will learn to focus instead on an entirely new goal - the energy you will gain...

Fixing your fatburn as fast and safely as possible, using all-natural foods and a few other metabolic 'hacks,' is the goal of this book."[51]

If you currently do not feel well when you have to eat a meal a few hours later than your usual time, Dr. Cate states that these feelings are likely because your metabolism is damaged. Irritability, nausea, fatigue, anxiety, and brain fog are symptoms of hypoglycemia, which do not normally happen if your metabolism is able to burn fat efficiently.[52]

The Diabetes Spectrum

Hypoglycemia is the first stage of what Dr. Cate calls "The Diabetes Spectrum." If you continue with unhealthy eating habits, this can lead you through the spectrum: hypoglycemia to insulin resistance to prediabetes and then to type 2 diabetes.[53] "Our ability to burn body fat is an underappreciated gift of nature and an unrecognized requirement for metabolic health that we almost never think about - until it starts to slip away."[54]

According to Dr. Cate, type 2 diabetes is not caused by an insulin deficiency but by an impaired metabolism.[55] She says that if you work on improving your fatburn, you will improve your metabolism and can prevent or even reverse type 2 diabetes.[56] In order to do this, *The Fatburn Fix* steers you away from starchy and sugary foods and allows you to be in control of what and when you eat.

5 Habits to Fix Your Fatburn

By reinforcing healthy habits and eventually restoring your metabolism, Dr. Cate states that you will not only start to have more energy but you will also see improvements in the way your hormones and organs (including your brain) function.[57] Within a few months of following her program, she states that most of her patients express how they have more energy to form new habits and no longer have to battle with hunger spells.[58] She also expresses that, "you will be vastly more able to achieve your potential," due to the cognitive benefits."[59]

The 5 habits/rules that Dr. Cate prescribes in *The Fatburn Fix* are:

1. Eat natural fats
2. Eat slow-digesting carbohydrates
3. Seek salt
4. Drink plenty of water
5. Supplement with vitamins and minerals[60]

Key Elements to Fix Your Fatburn

Fats, cholesterol, and salt are all things many people demonize but Dr. Cate argues that they are completely wrong. When it comes to fats, she explains how there are good fats and bad. An easy way to tell if a fat is natural or "good" is its taste. "All-natural fats have a lot of good flavor."[61] She also talks about how, unlike popular belief, cholesterol is not bad, whether it is LDL or HDL. High HDL has shown to be associated with greater memory, longevity, and IQ as well as decreased odds of dying from cancer or infection.[62] High LDL has been shown to be associated with increased longevity and decreased instances of dementia, infectious disease, and cancer. It can also be used as an indicator that you are burning more fat.[63]

Dr. Cate explains how salt can be used to help with energy, concentration, and digestion. She then suggests adding salt to as many meals as possible and if you need a snack, choosing something super salty, low-calorie, and healthy like a pickle or soup.[64] Another habit that she suggests is drinking at least eight glasses of water per day. This won't only curb your appetite but it will also help you with fixing your metabolism.[65]

Lastly, here are the vitamin and mineral supplement recommendations she provides for the purpose of helping you lose weight and fight inflammation:

- Magnesium oxide (250mg per day)
- Zinc picolinate (22mg per day)
- A daily multivitamin
- Vitamin D (2,000-4,000 IU per day)[66]

The Fatburn Fix Plan: Your Fat Quotient

After explaining the importance of fixing your metabolism and spelling out these five rules, Dr. Cate delves into the phases of The Fatburn Fix Plan. Before beginning, this program is designed to meet you where you are currently by figuring out your "Fat Quotient," which illustrates how efficiently you currently burn fat. She provides a quiz that takes into account your resting pulse, blood pressure, and fasting blood sugar as well asks questions like how often you feel tired, headaches, and heartburn. If you score a 20% on this quiz, that means your fatburning system operates at 20% capacity and if you score a 100%, your fatburn system is operating at 100% capacity.[67] The lower your score, the more time your body needs to reduce inflammation, repair your mitochondria and hormone sensitivity, and get rid of the toxins that are currently in your body fat.[68]

The Fatburn Fix Plan: Phase I

Dr. Cate states that if you currently feel you need to snack constantly, you will have to start with what she calls the "Baby Steps." If this is not the case for you and you can make it 1-2 weeks without feeling any mealtime hunger or hypoglycemia symptoms, you can start with what she calls the "Accelerated Plan." Both of these are part of Phase I of The Fatburn Fix Plan, which focuses on cutting out old habits and creating new ones that will improve how you feel.[69] To make it easier to cut out old habits, she states that you should think of it as switching one habit for another rather than giving something up.[70]

In Phase I, your two main goals are:

1. Stop snacking. Substitute snacks with non-caloric drinks like water, coffee, or unsweetened iced tea.
2. Avoid starchy and sugary foods. Have slow-digesting carbohydrates and clean-burning fats with each meal instead.[71] Dr. Cate states that eating more slow-digesting carbohydrates like beans, sourdough bread, and zucchini noodles rather than starchy carbohydrates like pasta, rice, and potatoes will help limit your carbohydrates and

smoothen the transition from a high-carb to a low-carb diet.[72] When people decide to drastically reduce carbohydrate intake immediately, she says this is why people get the low-carb/keto "flu."[73] In case you have not heard of this term before, this is where you do not feel well after starting to experiment with a low-carbohydrate diet.

The Fatburn Fix Plan: Phase II

Phase II of the program focuses on fasting and mindful eating. "Being in control of *when* you eat also helps you control *what* you eat."[74] Dr. Cate suggests using this phase for trying out new foods like kimchi, sushi, and canned fish[75] as well as experimenting with fasting. She strongly advises that you approach fasting carefully, starting out with one meal and attempting that once or twice a week.

Some experts suggest fasting for extended periods but she states that anything over 72 hours is overboard and you should only attempt multiple days in a row if you have been in Phase II for several months and have experimented enough to be comfortable with the idea. Many people also worry that fasting decreases muscle mass but she states that you should not worry about this if you are fasting for periods less than 72 hours at a time.[76]

Transitioning From High-Carb to Low-Carb

Whether you are in the Baby Steps of Phase I, the Accelerated Plan of Phase I, or Phase II, Dr. Cate provides meal plans and goes over substitutions to help transition from high-carb to low-carb.

She also gives suggestions for carbohydrate intake within each phase:

Phase I Baby Steps → <100g per day, or even <75g if possible[77]

Phase I Accelerated Plan → <50g per day[78]

Phase II → Switch it up. Some days, limit yourself to 20g and some days 70g (you can allow even more if you exercise).[79]

One of Dr. Cate's most prominent messages within this book is that most diets that are focused on weight loss actually damage our energy systems, which takes us down the slippery slope of The Diabetes Spectrum once we become reliant on sugar and don't realize we are overeating. Instead, this diet (which is implied to turn into a lifestyle) focuses on repairing the damage that has been done and providing you with the energy to reinforce good habits and create a "lasting relationship with healthy food."[80]

Conclusion

Dr. Cate's main objectives appear to be to explain things that are harmful to us and that most nutritionists ignore, like vegetable oils, and to show us how much our diet can influence our health as well as the health of generations to follow. On an interview with *Low Carb MD Podcast*, she states, "you are not your genes, [you are your genetic expression]" and "if there is anything that runs in your family disease-wise, that's not really a reflection of your genetic potential per se. It's a reflection of: How does the Standard American Diet cause disease in your family? And if you want to avoid disease, then that's where I want to help you."[81]

She guides us with achieving your true genetic potential and avoiding diseases of all kinds by fixing your fatburn, following her Four Pillars of World Cuisine, and eating a full range of real foods to get the nutrients your body needs. Dr. Cate has been working hard to influence as many people as possible: through her books, her involvement with sports teams like the LA Lakers and large companies like ABC Fine Wines & Spirits, her blog at *DrCate.com*, and her outreach through numerous events, television talk shows, and podcasts. "The last century has derailed our entire culture from the traditions that sustained us,"[82] and Dr. Cate has had the ambition to make a positive change in thousands of peoples' lives while continuing to expand her reach in order to get our health back on track.

More tips from Dr. Cate Shanahan:

- "Reorienting our financial priorities around healthy eating rebuilds our family's genetic wealth and is the best investment we can make."[83]
- "Grow a garden, shop for fruits and vegetables by smell (as opposed to appearance), and buy animal products from farms that raise them humanely - on pasture and outside in the sun."[84]
- Beauty and health are a package deal. Our diet can positively affect our body's symmetry, which in turn can prevent the need for glasses and braces as well as joint pain, sleep apnea, learning disorders, socialization disorders, cancers, and more.[85]
- Eating restaurant deep fried foods during pregnancy is likely to be as detrimental as smoking and drinking, if not moreso.[86]
- Milk has been shown to positively influence a child's height, especially during teenage years.
- Higher levels of omega-3 as a new-born has been shown to relate to a higher IQ on average later on as a child.[87]
- Insulin resistance in children has been shown to cause girls to form breasts at an early age and cause boys to have decreased penis sizes, muscle mass, and hair growth.[88]
- Going from a farming civilization to a city civilization negatively affected our bone structure. "You could say that, for the sake of developing agrarian civilizations, these societies chose to swap some of their vitality, toughness, and robusticity for aqueducts, large buildings, and other public works. Of course, if any group of people were to break away from city life and return to nomadic hunting or herding and gathering, they would... reclaim the physique they'd given up, their bodies would grow larger, and their skulls tougher and more robust."[89]
- "...vitamins manufactured in factories typically fail to approximate the real thing."[90]
- All natural, high-fat foods including corn, soybean, and sunflower seeds, are not harmful to eat. It's what happens during the process-

ing and refining along with the amount of processed oils we now consume that cause serious problems.[91]

- Heartburn is caused by gut inflammation and should be seen as a red flag that you need to change your diet. Frequent heartburn can potentially lead to damage to your body as well as your brain.[92]
- Cutting vegetable oil from your diet should be the first step if you are looking to improve your gut health because it will help you get rid of intestinal parasites and stomach inflammation.[93]
- Fish oil supplements are omega-3 oils that are very susceptible to being damaged. It is a better idea to get your omega-3s from real foods: grass-fed butter, nuts, sushi, green leafy vegetables, etc.[94]
- If you are a woman who suffers from migraines, you may be at high risk of having a stroke.[95]
- When a concussion occurs in a brain filled with fats that are susceptible to oxidation, like vegetable oils, that can lead to life-changing personality and mood changes. Since 30% of our brain is made up of these fatty acids and the brain is so delicate, you should remove vegetable oils from your diet in order to protect your brain, especially if you are an athlete.[96]
- Men are not off the hook when it comes to being healthy during conception. Dr. Cate states that men have been shown to influence the risk of autism in children and this is more of a worry nowadays because, "…according to new CDC statistics, it appears that autism rates have risen 30 percent between 2008 and 2012."[97]
- More research needs to be done to affirm this statement but one of Dr. Cate's hypotheses is that vegetable oil is the leading cause for the genetic mutations that lead to autism.[98]
- Exposure to lots of sugar as a child leads to chemical dependencies later on in life.[99]
- If you hunt, don't let anything go to waste if you know how to prepare it for eating.[100]
- Sprouted wheat bread is the healthiest bread you can buy. Many white flours are marketed as wheat - be sure to look for "whole wheat flour" to avoid falling for this trick. The next best thing is sourdough bread.[101]

- Not having enough body fat has been shown to have very similar effects as having too much body fat: blood clotting, negative effects on mood, concentration, and circadian rhythm.[102]
- Having a healthy body weight increases fertility and also helps ensure a happy pregnancy.[103]
- "I let all my patients suffering from depression in on a little secret: studies show that exercise is at least as effective as the best antidepressant medications."[104]
- "To get rid of cellulite, combine exercise with a diet full of healthy, natural fats (including animal fat) and collagen-rich stocks."[105]
- Vegetable oils make you more susceptible to being sunburnt and also to getting acne.[106]
- If you are not willing to try organ meats, eggs have similar nutritional benefits. You'll get the most nutrition by keeping the yolk runny.[107]
- "If you've already tried breaking the soda habit cold turkey and had no success, then I'd recommend trying these alternatives: ice-cold sparkling water with a lemon wedge, herbal tea, or 6 to 10 ounces of kombucha with the lowest amount of sugar you can find. I don't recommend diet soda unless you are using it as a bridge to kick the regular soda habit."[108]
- If you are a vegan, avoid oils and have plenty of nuts, avocados, and other natural fatty foods.[109]
- Rather than making a stop at a place like McDonalds, try to make it to the next meal instead if you don't have any healthy options or any options you like.[110]
- If you want to dramatically reduce your risk of food-borne illnesses, cook for yourself at home more often.[111]
- To avoid auto-immune diseases, steer clear of heavily processed foods, especially those high in protein.[112]
- One soda each day can increase your risk of a heart attack by 30% and increase calcium buildup in your arteries by 70%.
- If you are constipated, it is likely because of a lack of water or fiber. If that's not it, try using two tablespoons of ground flaxseed mixed in hot water.[113]

- If you have intestinal issues like indigestion or bloating, eat something acidic before meals that upset your stomach - for instance, try half a teaspoon of vinegar or a fermented pickle.[114] Drinking 2-3 cups of water with your meal can also help digesting certain foods.[115]
- Soy sauce will not hurt your health as long as it is fermented ('traditionally brewed') and not hydrolyzed.[116]
- Making smoothies with fruits and veggies is much more beneficial than juicing. The sugar stays but much of the nutrition is lost when juicing.
- Whether you are consuming sugar or artificial sweeteners like NutraSweet, Splenda, or stevia, your body reacts with insulin production which starts fat production.[117]
- "Breakfast is the most important meal of the day not to screw up." Rather than eating sugary, high-carbohydrate breakfast foods, eat high-fat foods like yogurt, smoothies, or eggs with avocado, non-starchy vegetables, and/or sausage. This will help you from being distracted by foods throughout the day and being hungry by lunch time.[118]
- Many of us overeat (by as much as 500-1,000 calories per day) and don't know it. [119] Keeping a daily food journal is a great way to see just how often you snack and how much you consume.[120]
- "Fortunately, the same diet that helps the body fight cancer also helps reverse diabetes: a high-fat ketogenic diet with intermittent fasting."[121]
- If you happen to have thyroid disease and thyroid hormone medications don't make you feel any better, improving your fatburn may help.[122]
- Ketones provide twice as much energy for the brain gram-per-gram than sugar does.[123] They also allow you to tolerate lower blood sugar levels[124] and generally make you smarter.[125] Sugar and protein shut down ketone production.[126]
- Some claim that you need to consume protein within thirty minutes after a workout to support muscle growth. This is not true. After a workout, you have a 24-48 hour window of muscle growth.[127]

- The later you eat carbohydrates, the less fat will build up.[128] Try to adopt the following limits: breakfast - 15g, lunch - 30g, dinner - 50g.[129]
- "If you are diabetic and take insulin or other drugs that lower your blood sugar, then going low-carb without knowing how to adjust your medications can put you at serious risk. When you cut your carbs, you reduce your need for insulin significantly."[130]
- Get three servings of dairy each day from different sources (milk, yogurt, cheese, etc.). If you don't, supplement with 250-500mg of calcium citrate.
- Cartilage and collagen supplements work great together if you don't eat enough meat on the bone. "Cartilage and collagen work together to support joint, hair, skin, and nail health, as well as gut health."[131]
- Many probiotic supplements are overhyped - eat natural foods for these if possible.[132]
- Rather than making a whole list of changes at once, try to make one new change each time you go to the market.[133]
- If you need help easing off of sugar, try this:

  * Limit yourself to one treat per day.
  * Reduce the sweetness of that treat (for example, switch from milk chocolate to dark chocolate).
  * Mix in slow-digestive carbohydrates and clean-burning fats with meals rather than having starchy and sweet foods.[134]

- If you are going to have fruit, berries and melons are your best options.[135]
- From worst to best - canned, frozen, or fresh veggies.[136]
- "If you don't have a steamer, the $30 investment will change your relationship with veggies forever."[137]
- To help curb hunger and cravings, there are a number of things that can help including: water, gum, or keeping yourself busy with a task, walk, or talk with a friend.[138]
- If you have a migraine or headache, it may be due to a lack of salt.[139]

- It is better to wait to eat after you exercise in order to maximize fatburn.[140]
- Dairy is maligned needlessly. Some arguments are a little silly. "People are the only animals to consume another species." So what? We're also the only animals to cook, write, and wear clothes. Other complaints against dairy come from misunderstanding, like the idea that dairy is inflammatory, for example. Compounds in milk stimulate mucus production in the GI tract in order to support the growth of beneficial bacteria. Some people will also develop upper airway mucus, but it's not an allergy or inflammatory process. It's just overly sensitive receptors.

Shared thoughts/ideologies:

- Shawn Stevenson states that we should use a different word than "fats" and use a nicer word like "lipids" so that we do not associate them directly with what causes fat to build up in our bodies. Dr. Cate takes it a step further and educates us on all of the different fats to separate good and bad fats:
    * Saturated fat, found in things like coconut oil, butter, and lard, assist our cells with generating energy. They also remain stable when heated so they are good to cook with.[141]
    * Monounsaturated fat, found in things like olive, peanut, and almond oil, also assist with our cells' energy production. They are relatively stable but have a low smoke point so should be stirred often when you are cooking with them.[142]
    * Polyunsaturated fat, found in things like vegetable oils as well as processed nuts and seeds, actually cause a decline in energy production.[143]
    * Trans fats, found in fried foods and dessert foods, are factory-made. They alter cell membranes and damage enzymes. If you see the word "hydrogenated" on a label, this should be a red flag that the product contains these toxic fats.[144]

- "Every bite you eat changes your genes a little bit."[145] Both Dr. Cate and Dr. Gundry believe that your health is not predetermined by your genes and that by eating a healthy diet, you can decrease your chances for all forms of disease and improve your family's genetic potential for the generations to come.
- Both Dr. Cate and Dr. Gundry state that most of today's fruits and vegetables are nutritionally bankrupt due to them being contaminated, modified, or picked too early. Both also say that vegetables are far healthier than fruits and organic is far better than the average fruit/vegetable.[146,147] Dr. Cate states that if you are on a budget, you should skip the organic fruits and vegetables and get the most important food when it comes to nutrition - properly raised animal products like grass-finished beef and grass-fed dairy.[148]
- Dr. Cate, Shawn Stevenson, and Ben Greenfield are all strong believers that, even though supplements can help, there is no substitute for real food.
- Both Dr. Cate and Ben Greenfield advocate buying from local farms, especially for meat.[149] They also share their love for organ meats and bone stock.
- Dr. Cate references the FASTER study regularly, which Ben Greenfield was involved in. Both of them believe strongly that more studies like this have to be done with fat-adapted athletes. The high-carbohydrate diet can't be called the "healthiest" or "best diet for athletes" until it is tested against subjects that are high-fat and truly fat-adapted, which can take months.
- Dr. Cate, Ben Greenfield, and Michael Matthews are all advocates for High Intensity Interval Training and reference similar studies showing their benefits. In *Deep Nutrition*, Dr. Cate highlights how HIIT can improve an athlete's exercise capacity/muscle power by 100% in just 2 weeks.[150]

Contradicting thoughts/ideologies:

- "Turns out, weight gain and weight loss isn't so much about energy as it is about *information*."[151] This goes against Mike Matthew's belief in energy balance. Dr. Cate does say calories *do* matter but emphasizes that real food is needed in order to "reshape your body and achieve maximum health."[152] In *Deep Nutrition*, she states that trans fats make us gain weight as well as dramatically increase our risk for insulin resistance and diabetes. In *The Fatburn Fix*, she points out that too much PUFA in our diet makes us hungry and tired. By avoiding foods like vegetable oils and margarines and instead eating foods like butter, cream, and coconut oil, food can actually help us get fit.[153]

- Dr. Gundry states that casein A2 is the healthier option over casein A1 (the type of milk that comes from most breeds of cows). Dr. Cate argues that this is not true and the *only* time casein A2 may be a better option is if you have an allergy to casein A1.[154]

If you know somebody who'd be interested in or could benefit from this book, tell them about it!

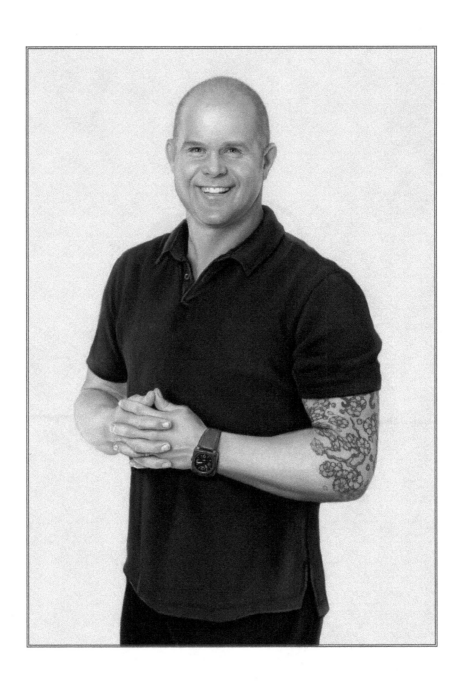

DR. KELLY STARRETT

"We're contending with a lot of the demands of being modern humans and it sets us up to not really reap the benefit and the bounty that is so extraordinary about being human. Because these bodies... They're badass, man."[1]

Kelly Starrett is an athlete, physical therapist, and (above everything else) strength and conditioning coach who focuses on movement. He has worked with athletes from several national and international teams including the Buffalo Bills, New York Giants, Golden State Warriors, New Zealand All Blacks, Toronto Blue Jays, and a variety of sports organizations like the NBA, MLB, NFL, NHL, and international Rugby as well as multiple (if not all) branches of the military. Kelly also coaches top-performing athletes one-on-one at his gym, San Francisco CrossFit, where he focuses less on volume and power and more on form and function being the keys to performance.

Kelly's wife, Juliet, is very much a partner in everything Kelly does: she is a lawyer by trade but also the entrepreneur behind and co-founder of the gym and their non-profit organization *StandUp Kids* as well as co-writer of Kelly's books. Never mind the fact that she is a three-time world champion, five-time national champion, and overall badass. Kelly and Juliet also have two kids together, Georgia and Caroline. Before continuing to Kelly's accomplishments, it is worth mentioning that many are Juliet's accomplishments as well.[2]

Kelly grew up in Garmisch, Germany, raised by a single mother. In multiple podcast interviews, he mentions how the culture he had growing up there was all about being as athletic as possible. He and his friends would ride their bikes everywhere, constantly competing and priding themselves on who was the least tired at the end of the day. He also competed at skiing at a young age.

Realizing the Relationship Between Pain & Sports

During his high school years, Kelly and his mom relocated to Colorado, where he started playing football but left that sport early on in college. Kelly then decided to take on Whitewater Kayak and Canoeing, which eventually led him to meeting Juliet as well as winning two national titles and appearing twice in the World Championships. After moving to San Francisco in 2000 and dealing with hand and knee pain from his football and whitewater slalom careers, he came to a realization while surfing that he wanted to pursue a career in physical therapy. Kelly went on to get a doctorate in Physical Therapy from Samuel Merritt University in 2008.

In a podcast interview for *PT Pintcast*, Kelly stated how he outworked his body into a hole and that the system was built on a model of what he calls "plausible deniability" - "if you outwork everyone and get hurt, it's not your fault." Kelly realized that it was not normal for men and women to have to deal with injuries constantly in order to continue in their sport and that he wanted to make his life's work into educating people on how they can help themselves with these issues.[3]

While Kelly was in college, he spent just as much time studying Olympic lifting/barbell training from coaches like Mark Rippetoe, Mike Bergener, and Jim Schmitz. Even though he had plenty of experience in specific sports, Kelly realized there was a big gap in his knowledge of strength training so he would visit their gyms and learn from them as often as possible.[4] When CrossFit had just started to surface, he took what he was learning and with Juliet started their own gym, San Francisco CrossFit. Now, San Francisco CrossFit has over fifteen coaches as well as four physical therapists to assist not only the top athletes but also the everyday people that show up there day after day.

The Three Categories of Strength Training

In *The Alpha Brew Podcast*, Kelly stated that when it comes to training, there are really three categories or ways to train:

1. General Physical Preparedness, or GPP, is working on foundational strength or fitness by practicing basic skills like push-ups and pull-ups.
2. Sports Preparation is mastering coordination and skill, like jumping and landing with your feet straight, to work on being able to pick up new sports and skills quickly.
3. Sports Specific Training is training skills for a specific sport so that you can be "good at your job" and/or be prepared. This means you are possibly sacrificing work in the other two categories.

The reason for having these categories are to know when you should be working on which area and to be aware of all the areas of strength training so that you can be a better athlete all-around.[5]

MobilityWOD/The 10-Minute Squat Test

After working with people for a few years in his gym, Kelly realized just how much work there was to be done. People were taking time off work to see him when they could be fixing these problems on their own by correcting their form and doing some soft tissue/mobility work. So in 2008, Kelly started his online program, MobilityWOD, giving people a Workout of the Day to assist them in accessing their full range of motion, correcting their form, and teaching them ways to fix stiff body parts and pain using tools like lacrosse balls, foam rollers, and compression bands. In 2012, MobilityWOD was named a Top 10 Fitness Blog by *BreakingMuscle.com*. At this time, Kelly committed himself to making a new video every day while also working at the gym open to close.

His most popular video is the first ever daily MobilityWOD video, which involved what he calls the 10-minute squat test. In this video, he guides you through an exercise that works on your ankle range of motion and reinforces keeping good form in this fundamental position. "Cultures that sleep on the ground see far less low back dysfunction, hip disease, and falls in older adults. The ability to get up and down from the floor is also a predictor of overall mortality. A Brazilian study showed that subjects who could not pass a simple test of getting up and down off the floor without support were more likely to die an early death. In other words, getting up and down off the floor is something you must practice regularly. Doing so will literally lengthen your life."[6]

Kelly highlights that you want to keep your heels on the ground, feet straight, and to use your hips to get up rather than your knees. The goal is to get ten total minutes all the way down in the squat position as if you were eating by a fire or taking a poop. He states that you should get up when/if you need to but to get right back down to accumulate the full ten minutes and if you need to hold onto something in the bottom position, that is okay too.

The Ready State

Videos are still being created on Kelly's YouTube channel regularly, showing a wide variety of helpful tips including: goal-setting, mobility exercises, strength exercises, and more. In 2019, after creating a log with thousands of videos and the term WOD becoming overused by others, Kelly and Juliet decided to rebrand MobilityWOD to another term that they use regularly,

The Ready State, to describe how their program helps keep you ready to perform at your highest level at all times.

On *TheReadyState.com*, it states that their program is founded on three founding principles:

1. It's impossible to reach your full potential if you're in pain, stiff, or tight.
2. Their work with elite athletes serves as the proving grounds for their methods.
3. Every human being should be able to perform basic maintenance on themselves.[7]

The third point is what Kelly emphasizes the most in interviews. As he states in the *Active Life Podcast* with Dr. Sean Pastuch, "doctors are experts in pathology and their experts in catastrophe. The rest of it belongs to us."[8] Even though Kelly has a lot of respect for (and also comes from multiple generations of) physicians, he explains that you should be able to realize why you have shoulder pain or knee pain, be able to manage the pain yourself, and correct the movement error that caused the problem in the first place to prevent the problem from happening again. "As we say: there's another step between the squat rack and the doctor's office. There's another step between the track and going to see the chiro; there has to be."[9] Kelly states that The Ready State program is most appropriate for coaches - teaching them to be able to evaluate dysfunction in their athletes and how to treat it as well as helping them find ways to improve their training programs.[10]

Kelly states that, "all good models are explanatory, predictive, repeatable. Create a model. Try and break it. Over and over. It should work across scale and cohort."[11] He also says how the gym should be looked at as a human performance laboratory for fixing movement inefficiencies and building skills. This means that you should not be training at the gym just so you can be better at the gym and it also means that it is not the place to perform maintenance on your body.[12] The Ready State program is meant to be done at home and is based on giving you access to all their past videos as well as new videos providing you with sessions that guide you whether you want to improve your form, relieve pain, or are looking for a pre-workout or post-workout exercise that are 10-15 minutes each.

Becoming a Supple Leopard

In combination with his online presence through his blog/mobility program and his flagship book, Kelly quickly became a well-known name throughout the fitness space. His flagship book, *Becoming a Supple Leopard*, was released in 2013 and made the New York Times and Wall Street Journal Bestseller lists. For four consecutive years (2013-2016), Kelly Starrett was listed in the Top 100 Most Influential in Health and Fitness by *Greatist.com* among names like Dr. Drew Pinsky, Gary Taubes, and Dr. Phil. *Becoming a Supple Leopard* continues to sell well (it is currently #18 in exercise and fitness books on *Amazon.com*) and is a staple book/manual for many coaches in either strength and conditioning or physical therapy.

"With enough practice, you can develop yourself to the point where your full physical capabilities are available to you instantaneously. You will develop the motor control and range of motion to do anything at any time. You could ultimately become the human equivalent of a supple leopard - always poised and ready for action. My system gives you the tools to dissolve the physical restrictions that are preventing you from fully actualizing your potential."[13] The start of this book provides what Kelly believes are the essentials for learning how to move correctly and how to be able to detect where you have limited range of motion. He teaches you what a stable position looks like versus a compromised position whether you are walking, sitting in a chair, or setting up to squat heavy. In these positions, the only major difference in your torso/trunk is how much you should be bracing your abdominals.

Stabilizing Your Spine

A common quote from Kelly (which is also used by Shawn Stevenson) is "practice makes permanent." Someone might argue that people sit slouched all the time or that they deadlift with extreme weights slightly hunched over and have not gotten injured but Kelly states that, even if you are not injured by this, "poor spinal mechanics lead to a host of biomechanical compromises and increase the potential for injury," and, "the way you do one thing is the way you do everything." In other words, you may be fine today, but something as simple as picking up your bags as you're leaving work can cause a tweak in your back simply because you have not taught yourself to get in the habit of bracing your spine correctly.[14]

Torque

Once Kelly teaches you to stabilize yourself in good positions, he highlights the importance of torque during movements. By utilizing torque, he states that this forces your body to stay in good position and have better consistency in repetitions. For instance, if you twist the inside of your elbows outwards while doing a push-up, it will keep your elbows from flaring out and if you push your knees outwards while doing a squat, it will keep your knees from going inwards which could cause knee pain.[15] "When both of these factors are in proper alignment, meaning that your trunk is organized and you're applying the right amount of torque through your joints, your ability to generate maximum force - safely and without risk of injury - improves dramatically."[16]

Assessing Your Range of Motion

Following these principles, Kelly lays out the basic configurations that he calls "the seven archetypes," which are the start and/or end positions of most movements and covers full range of motion (mainly in your shoulders, hips, and ankles). These seven archetypes include overhead, press, hang, front rack, squat, pistol, and lunge. "If you can express competency in these positions, you have the building blocks to create safe, stable positions for most movements."[17] Kelly provides simple tests like putting your arms overhead, doing push-ups correctly, and hip-hinging correctly and then explains how to use these tests as diagnostic tools to figure out where you have limited range of motion.

Along with having full range of motion in these seven positions, he believes that our bodies are designed to be able to do certain movements, therefore every adult should be able to do them.[18] Here are some examples:

- "We have a saying around our gym: Your shoulders are abnormal unless you can jerk."[19] If you are unfamiliar with this term, search 'the press jerk CrossFit' on YouTube to see demonstrations.
- "…You need to be able to pick up heavy, awkward objects and not mess up your back. It's part of being a fully functional human being."[20]
- "Bending and squatting are natural movements that all of us should be able to perform efficiently."[21]

Improving Your Movement

Kelly also shows you how to achieve proper form in these basic configurations so that you can do what he calls Category 1 Movements like the squat, deadlift, bench press, and pull-up in a safe manner. Category 2 Movements add more movement and break the position at some point, like during a kettlebell swing or when jumping and landing. Category 2 Movements still only involve one archetype while Category 3 Movements start in one archetype and end in another, like during a snatch, clean, or muscle up.

"I realized by systematically progressing movements - from basic to more advanced - I could not only rehab an injured athlete, but also build efficient movement patterns in both novices and elites."[22] On a podcast interview for *The Tim Ferriss Show*, Kelly talks about how at San Francisco CrossFit, athletes often work with PVC pipes for more complicated movements like the clean to ensure they have proper form before picking up the barbell and adding weight.[23]

After testing your movements and finding where you can improve your mobility, Kelly provides over 150 pages of techniques in *Becoming a Supple Leopard* that you can use to "help you address short and tight muscles, soft tissue and joint capsule restriction, motor control problems, and joint range of motion limitations."[24]

Mobility/Pain Relief Tools & Exercises

Kelly suggests starting out using tools like foam rollers and yoga tune up balls before moving up to the more painful lacrosse balls, softballs, and compression bands. He even suggests using barbells and kettlebells to smash your knotted tissues once you get comfortable enough.

Generally, the more rigid the ball is, the more effective it will be at improving your mobility. Balls are mainly used for three methods that Kelly describes in *Becoming a Supple Leopard*:

1. **Pressure Wave**

    Roll on the ball until you find a tight muscle or knot. Then, sink that area of your body into the ball and slightly roll on that area with your bodyweight. Take deep breaths to sink in. Stay relaxed on the ball and move slow. This is mainly used to resolve soreness/tightness.[25]

2. **Contract and Relax**

    Put a body part into end range of motion and hold that in place for five seconds. Then, release the tension and then move that body part into a further end range and stay there for at least ten seconds. This is mainly used to improve range of motion and muscle contraction.[26]

3. **Smash and Floss**

    Find the tightest, most knotted muscle areas and put as much pressure as possible on that area by putting a ball between that body part and a rigid surface. Then, move that body part and body parts that are closely connected in full range of motion in every direction. This is mainly used to loosen up the tissue and restore sliding surfaces.[27] Take long, deep breaths so that your muscles can relax while smashing.[28]

Kelly generally suggests using these methods post-workout or before bed because they will help you relax. Bands, on the other hand, are generally suggested before a workout. He states that wrapping resistance bands around limbs while doing movements and flossing is "one of the best ways to prepare for dynamic or loaded movements."[29] Kelly mainly uses resistance bands to improve range of motion or to fix an impingement in joint capsules like in the hip.

Compression bands are a much different tool and are mainly used to work on a swollen or painful area. Kelly suggests using compression bands if you have a swollen ankle or are treating things like tennis elbow. This is an intense tool and needs to be done properly and safely - you are partially restricting blood flow in those painful areas and putting them into their full range of motion.[30]

Lastly, one of the most effective tools that Kelly suggests is employing what he calls a "Superfriend." The Superfriend is another person that, once you are in the correct position and you have agreed to a safe word, carefully puts pressure on your muscle using their feet - from your feet to your calves and from there to your quads and your triceps, to name a few. Keep in mind, even though these tools and methods may sound strange, Kelly has tested and retested this systematic approach and they have shown to be effective.

Whether you have pain in your lower back, hip, or knee, or you want to work on your mobility so that you can perform movements with correct form, or you just feel like your work or personal life does not provide you with the movement you need to keep your joints healthy, Kelly has prescriptions for you that can be found in *Becoming a Supple Leopard* and he also shows you how to create your own plan based on your lifestyle and goals. "As long as you're putting in the daily maintenance, you will experience long-term change."[31]

Deskbound: Standing Up to a Sitting World

Kelly has followed *Becoming a Supple Leopard* up with multiple successful books, including *Ready to Run* in 2014, *Deskbound* in 2016, and then *Waterman 2.0* in 2018. These books are similar to *Becoming a Supple Leopard* but dig deeper into the associated activities/lifestyles. *Deskbound: Standing Up to a Sitting World*, for example, is not only about those with desk jobs but is a counter to the sedentary lifestyle that most of us adopt due to the fact that Americans sit for an average of 13 hours per day between our car rides to and from work, at our desk at work, sitting at every meal, watching TV at home, etc.[32] Kelly takes this very seriously, stating that we are starting to see, "the wholesale de-evolution of the human being," due to the lack of movement in our lives. The goal of *Deskbound* is to explain how adding movement to your life can not only improve your health but also your overall quality of life.[33]

StandUp Kids

Even before the release of *Deskbound*, Kelly and Juliet created a movement of popularizing standing desks. In 2012, they converted their office into a standing office and in 2013, they volunteered at their daughters' field day at school and realized they needed to do something bigger. Not only did they notice the number of overweight kids but they also noticed that the kids could not move well - they were not able to do the sack race because they lacked the range of motion.

In 2014, the movement started and their daughter's fourth grade classroom had been converted to a standing classroom thanks to their discussion with the principal. By the end of 2015, the rest of Vallecito Elementary School was converted to standing classrooms thanks to Kelly and Juliet's work with StandUp Kids, their non-profit organization with the powerful goal of converting all public schools to standing desks by educating schools and donors.

Kelly and Juliet have been speaking out and fighting against schools doing things like taking away PE programs, having soda in vending machines, and loading kids with sugar during sports. Instead, they encouraged movement-rich classrooms and as much playtime as possible. Kelly has realized by talking to kids at schools as well as coaches of all levels (from high school to collegiate to professional) that movement dysfunction needs to be addressed as early as possible, ideally in elementary and middle school. He states how as early as the first grade, kids start heel striking when running which is known to cause problems later if it is not addressed.[34]

The Negative Aspects of Sitting Too Much

In multiple interviews, Kelly expresses how StandUp Kids is his and Juliet's life's work that they are most proud of. The research that Kelly shares in *Deskbound* is profound and is mainly done by Mark Benden. Mark is an associate professor and department head for the Department of Environmental and Occupational Health as well as Director of the Ergonomics

Center for the Texas A&M School of Public Health. He is also a researcher, speaker, and a prominent writer on topics like optimizing productivity in call centers, the negative effects of sedentary behavior, and standing desks.

Here are some of the most eye-opening facts and statistics mentioned in *Deskbound*:

- "A British study of more than 4,000 civil servants found that spending less than 12 hours a week sitting decreased diabetes risk by 75 percent. Those who sat more than 25 hours a week had an increased chance of developing metabolic risk factors like diabetes, insulin resistance, and 'bad' cholesterol."[35]
- A study done by UC Berkeley showed, "for every hour that children ages 12 to 17 sit watching TV, their likelihood of being overweight increases by 2 percent."[36]
- "Today, the World Health Organization ranks physical inactivity - sitting too much - as the fourth biggest preventable killer globally, causing an estimated 3.2 million deaths annually. In the past 20 years, the simple act of sitting has leapfrogged to the top of the health killer charts globally... Unless we are asleep, we human beings are designed to move."[37]

The Benefits Seen from Standing Desks

Not all of the research is negative. The results from replacing sedentary desks with standing desks has shown things like decreases in BMI in schoolchildren and increases in productivity in classrooms and profit in call centers.[38] Debatably, the most interesting are the increases in cognitive function. Physical activity has been shown to increase the volume of gray matter in the basal ganglia and hippocampus, the parts of the brain related to cognitive control and memory. It has also been shown to increase BDNF (brain-derived neurotrophic factor), which optimizes your brain for learning - allowing you to stay sharp, focus more, and enhance your mental circuits. Any brain benefits are especially impactful for children while their brains are in development.[39]

Throughout *Deskbound*, Kelly explains how converting your workstation to a standing desk and moving more during the day reduces your risks of diabetes, high cholesterol,[40] obesity, and heart disease[41] while improving memory[42] and learning capabilities (especially in children with ADHD).[43] Even with high-profile athletes looking to reduce their risk of injuries, Kelly prescribes standing and moving more outside of practice because a couple hours of training does not make up for consecutive hours spent sitting.[44]

Hire a Friend

Kelly's principles remain the same by first teaching us to value positions and mechanics and then encouraging 10-15 minutes of daily maintenance. He recommends having both someone at work and someone at home to address when they notice that your posture is less than optimal.[45] By sitting in a slouched position, he explains how we are not only compromising our spine but also our glutes, pelvis, and shoulders which, in turn, leads to a loss in a range of motion, weakened breathing, numbness/tingling in our arms and hands, headaches, and pain in our neck, shoulders, lower back, and jaw.[46]

Foot Care

By wearing shoes with an elevated heel or that are tight on your feet, Kelly explains that your spine has to compensate by overextending. When you wear tight shoes or shoes with a lot of cushion, you are slowly losing ankle range of motion due to improper walking mechanics. He understands that high heels and dress shoes are needed on occasion but says that you should be aware of the negative effects and encourages being as close to barefoot as you can, as much as possible. Just as he recommends keeping your feet straight when squatting, he also states that you should focus on keeping your feet straight whether you are walking around the office or at your standing desk to avoid problems like tight calves and weak heels or ankles. "The bottom line is that your feet are the foundation for your entire body… Compromised feet set off a chain of problems that ultimately work their way up the whole kinetic chain."[47]

Adjusting to Your Standing Desk

Kelly commonly says that you do not have a standing workstation until you have a place to put your feet. By adding a rail, slant board, or the like to rest your foot on, you will find it much easier to stand for hours at a time. Next, he asks that you position the top of the monitor to be eye level and to position your keyboard so that your forearms are parallel with the floor and that your elbow makes a 90° angle between your bicep and forearm. Lastly, he encourages having a stool, more to lean on than for sitting.[48]

"The fact that standing is strenuous is a sign that your body is out of whack, because the human body is designed to be upright and moving."[49] Nonetheless, Kelly states that it will likely take about six weeks to transition to the standing desk and the key to a smooth transition is movement. He explains that your body will likely get tired from standing in this transition period, but recommends not sitting for any longer than twenty minutes at a time.[50] Standing is the better option than sitting because of the fact that it adds more movement options so Kelly provides several position options. He also encourages taking a break to move every 20-30 minutes. Taking a break to walk around is not only good for your body, but also allows you to engage and focus more when you return to your work.[51]

Mobility Work at Your Desk

For mobility work related to anyone that is deskbound, Kelly prescribes exercises that open up your neck, wrists, hips, quads, shoulders, chest, glutes, hips, forearms, and feet. Most of these mobilizations do not involve any tools and are basic movements like the squat or rolling your wrists but some involve a lacrosse ball (which you could easily keep at your desk) to smash your forearms, quads, feet, etc.[52]

Lifestyle Practices

As important as Kelly believes mechanics and daily mobility work are, in *Deskbound*, he calls out another piece of the puzzle - lifestyle. "We support the idea that small consistent lifestyle changes can aggregate to significantly improve overall health."[53] He spells out how your sleep, hydration/nutrition, and exercise (along with good mechanics) all need to be optimal in order to live a long, movement-rich life and to minimize injury. All of these elements together are what Kelly calls your "physical practice."

Exercise

For the exercise component of your physical practice, Kelly is not partial to any particular activity, whether it be Pilates, yoga, CrossFit, just lifting weights, or something else. He states that exercising on a regular basis will not only prepare you for your sport but also make you less susceptible to overall pain. Kelly commonly says in podcast interviews that it is amazing how much our bodies can withstand but he highly encourages having a physical practice because the better you take care of your body, the better off you'll be.

For everyday movement, Kelly believes that the common 10,000 steps/day rule should be followed as the "minimum therapeutic dose". He and Juliet started a walking school bus, where parents drop off their kids or walk along with them a mile and a half each morning to get to school. On *The Model Health Show* with Shawn Stevenson, Kelly explains how he had a parent say that they lost twenty pounds by taking part in the walking school bus and uses that as an example to show that our body craves this basic input.[54] A common thread in *The Ready State Podcast* between Kelly, Juliet, and their good friends like Laird Hamilton and Dr. Mark Benden is that the people they know who are age 75 or older and can still move well have simply always been movers.[55]

The Ready State Podcast

The Ready State Podcast was a project started by Kelly and Juliet in 2018 to capture conversations they have with friends and people who have had heavy influence on their thinking on topics like longevity, nutrition, pain, CrossFit, and children's sports practices. For example, they talk to their good friend and surfing legend Laird Hamilton on overcoming pain through the number of injuries he has had to overcome while continuing to be a top-performing surfer. They also talk to Matt Hasselback, a well-known quarterback who spent eighteen seasons in the NFL and now commentates for ESPN, about longevity and how the NFL's practices have changed over the years. Other professional athletes and experts/friends that they interview, among many, include George St. Pierre, Alex Hutchinson, Mike Burgener, and Dr. Cate Shanahan.

Nutrition

Kelly's outlook on nutrition is strongly influenced by Dr. Cate Shanahan - stating that you should be vegan in the sense that you are eating as many organic vegetables as you possibly can each day but also suggests eating the best quality meat (grass-fed and free-range) on the bone. He says that we should strive to reach 800 grams of fruits and vegetables each day, which is influenced by a challenge started by EC Synkowski of OptimizeMe Nutrition. If people come to Kelly with issues, the first thing he addresses is their physical practice. If their tissues feel weak or stiff, he ensures their moving, eating, and (most important of all) sleeping well before jumping into physical therapy practices.

Hydration

Kelly believes that staying hydrated is important, but suggests not to overdo it. On *The Bulletproof Radio Podcast* with Dave Asprey, he recalls how he met a 120lb diva working with the WWE who stated that she drank a gallon and a half of water per day. His response was, "you're drinking enough water for like a 350lb guy in the middle of the NFL," and follows it with a recommendation that women who exercise should have a goal of 2 liters of water per day and 3 liters per day for men who exercise.[56] Kelly also recommends adding a pinch of salt to your water because this allows you to absorb the water you drink, keeping you more hydrated while reducing the number of trips to the bathroom and chances that you will pee yourself.[57] He says that this trick also improves the health of your tissues so it is also beneficial for those with arthritis.[58]

Sleep

In interviews, whenever Kelly is asked for a tip that he has for everyone, he makes sure to bring up how he and his family work hard to protect their sleep. Kelly's goal is to be in bed by 10:00 p.m. every day and ensures that he sleeps in a room that is between 62-68 degrees Fahrenheit and has no light whatsoever.[59] Him, Juliet, and his daughters all lock their phones in a box before heading to bed to make sure the blue light and all the distractions on their phones do not mess with their sleep. Even for elite athletes, Kelly states that sleep is the first thing he examines and he recommends Matt Walker's book, *Why We Sleep* or Shawn Stevenson's *Sleep Smarter*.

The Importance of Moving Daily

On *The Model Health Show*, Kelly relates having a daily physical practice to sport by saying:

> "...this is why we do sport in the first place. Not to win Olympic medals, not to be on a team for any other reason than it helps us know ourselves, and it helps us know our friends, and it helps us see the world very cleanly, and I think this is why I hope that everyone has some kind of competitive, or at least a physical practice, because it really simplifies in a really easy model what's working in your life and what's not working in your life."

He states that we need to focus on first principles. After talking about sleep, the second thing he looks at is movement throughout the day and ways athletes can add more walking into their lives. Then, this opens the conversation for vegetables, coffee, kettlebells, deadlifting, and other training basics.[60]

Ready to Run & Waterman 2.0

On a podcast interview for *The Fat Burning Man* with Abel James, Kelly says that his books *Ready to Run* and *Waterman 2.0*, which were released in

2016 and 2018 respectively, tell us why those activities are important, what we can improve in the activities we love, and also what we can do to prevent injuries so that we are able to do those sports for longer. *Ready to Run* clearly focuses on running while *Waterman 2.0* focuses on watersports like the sport he is most passionate about, paddling. He also mentions a book that he has been working on, *Flight Plan*, which will tell us how we can take care of ourselves to perform at our best when dealing with airplane travel.[61]

Conclusion

For the past decade, Kelly has been working hard to teach coaches, athletes, and everyday people how to improve their lives by working on their physical practices. By being transparent and sharing his thoughts and experiences through books, podcasts, keynote speeches, and in his own gym, he has become a strong force in the health and fitness space. You can even still see Kelly's first blog, *sanfranciscocrossfit.blogspot.com* that shows the community that Kelly built and his dedication to improve the fitness world. Every day through YouTube and *TheReadyState.com*, Kelly continues to add to his endless pool of content with the goal to help anyone who is looking for a virtual coach. "The bottom line is that you can always improve and be working towards positive change. You just have to remain consistent and implement the right practices… And never take a day off."[62]

The bottom line is that Kelly has been a fantastic example of how we can, as he says in volleyball terms, "improve the ball." Not only how to improve yourself but also the people around you by doing things like leading a walking school bus each morning, opening your home as a community gym, or even creating communities like San Francisco CrossFit, starting with your friends and then taking what you know and impacting the world in a positive way by doing things like inspiring people you work with or schools you are involved with to incorporate standing desks. Little by little, Kelly has worked his way to making a big impact on millions of people, young and old. He is an impactful leader in the health and fitness realm and I'm sure he still has plenty of wisdom to share and an even bigger influence to make.

More tips from Dr. Kelly Starrett:

- To avoid an unfavorable neck/jaw position while lifting, jam your tongue against the roof of your mouth behind your teeth and then close your mouth.[63]
- One simple way to avoid the negative effects of sitting for long periods is by standing and reorganizing yourself every 10-15 minutes. You can also just switch positions as often as possible (pick certain positions for certain tasks or set a timer to give yourself a reminder).[64]
- Compromising your posture forces weak breathing patterns that negatively affect multiple areas of your life including performance, sleep, and recovery.[65]
- The joint you move first will carry the bulk of the load during that movement.[66]
- Your hips and shoulders are what Kelly calls your "primary engines." During movements, distribute as much weight through your hips and shoulders rather than through joints like your knees or elbows.[67]
- Spreading your legs while doing a pushup is not optimal because it makes it more difficult to clench your stomach and glutes.[68]
- "If you don't start right, you won't finish right. And if you don't finish right, your next position will be compromised."[69] If you find yourself in a bad position, start over and instill good position before continuing.
- You need a coach to assist you in scaling your capabilities up and down. Coaches and training partners are also needed to hold you accountable by reinforcing good positions and movement patterns.[70]
- Don't just listen to your strength and conditioning coach or physical therapist. Seek out experts of assorted fields to find what works best for you.[71]
- If you want to fix tight muscles or develop motor control and strength, exercise to the full extent of the movement. For example, getting to the bottom of a squat will help with tight hamstrings

and will extend and strengthen your leg muscles. Then, add load to increase the benefits.[72]

- If you have pain or lack range of motion in an area, don't just focus on that muscle but also mobilize the areas above and below.[73]
- Develop a list of problem areas that you want to improve and work on those areas for a portion of your daily mobility work.[74]
- If something feels painful or wrong while doing mobility work, don't push through it because you will likely make that pain worse and possibly injure yourself. "Stand at the entrance of the pain cave but do not enter the pain cave. Mobility should be uncomfortable but not unbearable." Some find a glass of wine can help make mobility work more bearable (but don't go overboard).
- Don't take any days off from mobilizing, even if you take the day off from the gym. This will keep muscles from getting stiff and sore as well as prepare you for the next time you need to work out or play.[75]
- For an optimal squat position for most people, follow these rules:

  * Position your feet slightly past your shoulders.
  * Keep your shins as vertical as you can.
  * Carry the weight in your hamstrings and hips.[76]
  * If you struggle to squat your butt below knee-level, practice your mechanics by placing a box or chair around knee level behind you.[77]

- "People who understand how to deadlift with good form… typically have fewer back problems."[78]
- Performing a push-up with your knees on the ground prohibits you from squeezing your butt and creating full tension in your trunk. If you have trouble with push-ups, try raising the level your hands are on or wrapping a large band from elbow to elbow.[79]
- Rings are a great tool for improving your mechanics for movements like push-ups and dips because they force good position, stable shoulders, and a stable trunk.[80]
- Coaches working with athletes that do overhead movements often like volleyball players, swimmers, or baseball pitchers should implement movement exercises that train the overhead and press

positions like the push-up and strict press to train and test shoulder stability in end-range positions.[81]

- If possible, it is best to use a barbell for loaded overhead movements because it is easier to get in position with good form.[82]

- "If you're an average person, the handstand pushup is a fundamental skill that will improve your athleticism and, more important, will tell you a lot about your ability to organize your shoulders and trunk in an unfamiliar position."[83]

- Pull-ups do a better job of teaching good shoulder position, trunk stabilization, and torque than chin-ups so learn proper pull-ups before working on chin-ups.[84]

- "Reconstruct the workout so that it rewards athletes for their movement quality, not for finishing with the fastest time. For example, you could pair them up and have one person perform a set number of burpees in a row while her partner silently counts a point for every fault she commits. The goal is to get the lowest score possible."[85]

- If you have lower back pain, it will not get any better unless you fix your position and perform maintenance on that area of your body.[86]

- Smash your diaphragm at least once a week. "When your respiratory diaphragm is stiff, your breathing is compromised."[87]

- "Just remember, the more uncomfortable the mobilization, the more change you will see, feel, and realize."[88]

- "We've never met an arch that we couldn't reclaim.[89] Most [foot] arches can be restored within a year but the problem needs to be addressed consistently and you need to be patient."[90]

- If you can't afford a standing desk or want to test it out, you can make one by placing your monitors on cardboard boxes.[91] Boxes, chairs, and balls could also be used in place of a rail or slant board.[92]

- If you are not able to get a standing desk, move around for at least 2 minutes every half hour.[93]

- Sitting on the ground is always better than sitting on the couch - and while you are watching TV on the ground, work on your mobility.[94]

- Breathing through your nose allows you to relax muscles from your neck to your jaw and face as well as breathe deeper and longer than breathing through the mouth.[95]
- Keeping your abs in low tension (at about 20%) while standing and walking around will allow you to keep an organized spine and will help you stay ready for your next movement.[96]
- Try to be barefoot as much as possible - this will help with balance, posture, and strengthening your lower body.
- Keep flat shoes (not flip flops) beneath your desk so you can switch out of your dress shoes or heels while you are at your workstation.[97]
- When you go to pick something up, the most efficient method is to get the object as close to your feet as you can before squatting down/hinging over.[98]
- Turning your palms up is an easy way to get your shoulders in the right position. When you feel yourself slouching your shoulders, take a second to readjust using this trick.[99]
- Make sure the surface you are standing on at your workstation has just enough cushion to stand comfortably for hours at a time. Add cushion with lightly cushioned shoes or an anti-fatigue mat if needed.[100]
- To prevent staring at a screen from weakening your eyes, use what Kelly calls the 20-20-20 rule: every 20 minutes, stare at an object 20 feet away for at least 20 seconds.[101]
- Take frequent breaks to move your wrists and keep your wrists parallel with your forearms when you are typing.[102]
- When you are transitioning to the standing desk, consider standing for certain tasks and sitting for others (use standing for the tasks that require more time).[103]
- Sit on the edge of your seat in order to stay in good position, keeping your trunk tight and your weight centered over your hips.[104]
- "Our advice: LISTEN TO YOUR BODY... When your body sends you the signal to move, stand up and reset your position."[105]
- The only time Kelly suggests using lumbar support is when you are forced to sit for a long period of time, like during airplane travel. Position the back support whether it be a pillow, towel, jacket, or

inflatable pad at either the base of your rib cage or just beneath your belt line.[106]

- Wear compression socks when you are expected to sit for long periods, like when traveling on an airplane or when you know you have a long meeting. This helps your circulatory and lymphatic systems as well as helps you avoid swollen ankles.[107]
- When you are taking long trips, whether in a car or on a plane, take movement breaks as much as you can. If you pull over at a rest stop, take some time to stretch. Also, as soon as you reach your destination, do 10-15 minutes of mobility work.[108]
- Most adults need between 7-9 hours of sleep each night.[109]
- If you do not want to use electrical tape to create a pitch-black room to sleep in, consider using a sleep mask.[110]
- If you have back pain, begin walking more to restore function.
- If you have a little kid at home and a free day on the weekend, do everything your kid does. Toddlers walk an average of 2.5 miles per day. You'll find you won't have to warm up as much and you'll be able to maintain a normal range of motion simply by being human and staying in motion.[111]
- If you are in your mid 30s or older, use less complicated movements and add heavy cardio between sets. For example: between sets of squats, row 1,000m or between sets of floor pressing, bike 3-5 minutes and get your heart rate going. This will help you be less sore after exercising at a high volume.[112]
- If you can spend multiple days consecutively without shoes (especially outdoors), you'll find your feet are stronger and you'll be more ready to run.[113]
- Treat alcohol as a dessert and not as something you do every day. Also, avoid alcohol in times of stress.
- Avoid caffeine after 4:00 p.m. If you are sensitive to caffeine, avoid it after 12:00 p.m.[114]

Shared thoughts/ideologies:

- Kelly and Shawn Stevenson believe strongly in the saying, "practice makes permanent." Not only do good practices reinforce good practices in the future but by constantly making bad decisions, you'll see that they pile up. "If you sit, stand or walk with an overextended or rounded back, chances are you will have trouble organizing your spine in a good position during loaded or dynamic athletic movements. The best defense is not to make those errors in the first place."[115]

- Kelly, Ben Greenfield, and Michael Matthews all agree that static stretching is not the right way to warm up for an exercise. "Stretching is not the answer. Instead you need to deal systematically with each of the problems that are preventing you from getting into ideal positions and moving correctly."[116]

- Kelly and Michael Matthews agree that while volume is important in the gym, you should never sacrifice form.

- Kelly and Mike use the term "break the bar" as a cue when you are gripping a barbell during a bench press in order to get the best grip and torque on the bar and to keep your shoulders and elbows in good position.[117]

- Kelly, Shawn, and Ben all have similar recommendations when it comes to protecting your sleep by keeping your room cool and dark as well as by avoiding blue light. In *Deskbound*, Kelly suggests turning off bright screens 2-3 hours before bedtime and using things like blue light-blocking glasses or software to deter the bright lights from negatively affecting melatonin production at night time.[118]

- Kelly, Shawn, Ben, Dr. Gundry, and Dr. Cate all agree that we should look for grass-fed, free-range, and organic products because they are more nutrient-dense than foods that do not have these labels.[119]

Contradicting thoughts/ideologies:

- Kelly is a strong proponent for exercising with your feet as straight as possible, never suggesting pointing your feet out past 12° during a squat. This goes against Mike Matthew's advice of squatting with your feet turned out between 20-25°.[120] Kelly states that once you get towards 30 degrees, you lose the capability of using torque and you are also instilling a bad movement pattern.[121] He also says that keeping your feet straight will give you better support and balance.[122]

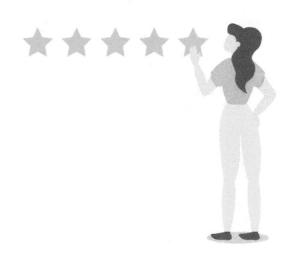

If you've enjoyed this book, the best way to show support is to take a minute and go leave a review on Amazon.com.

Please and thank you! ☺

CONCLUSION/THANK YOU

The fact that you've made it this far says something about you. It means that you care enough about yourself or your clients to further your knowledge beyond what you learn in school or from your own experiences. Today, we have access to an endless amount of information from people who sincerely just want to help as many individuals as possible and my goal is to show you some of the people who do that best. I hope that after reading those biographies, you found one or two experts who you decided to follow whether by reading their books, listening to their podcasts, watching their YouTube Channels, or trying out their programs.

The amount of research done to provide you with this information was something like 400+ hours of listening, 4,000+ pages of reading (but who's counting), and who knows how many blog articles I read and hours spent on trying out programs. My highest hopes are that you found something of value from each of these experts to change your life for the better and that you found an expert or two that you'll continue to follow.

I sincerely want to thank you for taking the time out of your busy life to read this book. If you have any questions or comments, you can always email me at jake@inspiringleaderscollective.com. I always read and respond to my emails personally (I apologize if it takes me a week or so).

You can also find me at:

www.InspiringLeadersCollective.com – A site dedicated to this book series

www.TwelvePaths.com – My personal blog site

If you enjoyed this book, I have one quick favor to ask. The best thing that you can do to support this book and my work in general is to go review this book on Amazon.com. Please go to Amazon.com, search for "Inspiring Leaders in Health & Fitness," click on the book, scroll down until you see the section with reviews, and click on the button that says, "Write a customer review."

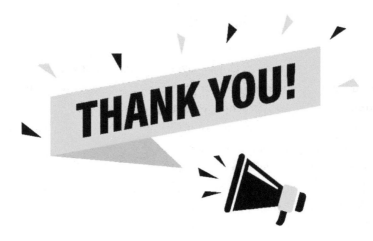

Thank you again and be on the lookout for the next book! ☺

ACKNOWLEDGEMENTS

Through the process of getting this book complete, there are two very important lessons that I learned (amongst many):

1. If I think a book will take 1 year to research, write and self-publish, it will take at least 2 if I work my tail off.
2. The word 'self-publish' is deceiving.

Although I am sure traditional publishing is much more stressful because of how many things are out of your control, self-publishing a book is not a simple task by any means and it can't be done alone. It takes a team.

From proofreaders to beta readers to editors, from artists to graphic designers to website designers, other authors willing to offer help or who helped me through their books, the leaders that I reached out to that responded and offered helpful advice, and friends, family, and fans who simply showed support along the way - they were all an important part of the process.

To everyone who gave their bit of support - I cannot thank you enough for taking the time out of your busy life to help me make this book a reality.

To Olayiwola Janet Oluwatobiloba (editor), Natalya Kopylova (portrait artist), Qamar Sultan (graphic designer), Myrah Summers (medical writer of the Foreward), Josh Rapps (References editor), Roggo and the team at *99designs.com* (logo design for book series), and Chrissy and the team at

Damonza.com (book cover and interior formatting) for assisting me with improving the quality of this book and setting the stage for my book series with your amazing work and hard efforts.

To Michael Hyatt, Karl Palachuk, Stephanie Chandler, Gundi Gabrielle, and Alexandra Watkins for assisting me through the process with your books.

To my girlfriend, Taylor, my parents, Greg and Christine, Angela Livinlyf, Robyn Vicaire, Uncle Craig, Wendell Butler, Catherine Kaiser, Michael Reynolds, Aunt Carole, Mrs. Heflin, and the rest of my team of beta readers for going above and beyond with your support.

To all of the leaders I've reached out to who responded with feedback and additional support, including: Ben Greenfield, Michael Matthews, Dr. Cate Shanahan, and Greg Nuckols.

To leaders like Jocko WIllink and Eric Thomas who sparked the inspiration to get this journey started for me.

I'm sure there's somebody that I missed that I'll soon feel bad I forgot to mention and additional people who assisted after writing this. Please know how much I appreciate your help creating this book. It was a heck of a process but we did it.

FREE BONUS MATERIAL

Visit
www.InspiringLeadersCollective.com

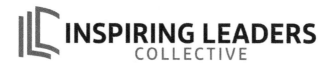

www.TwelvePaths.com

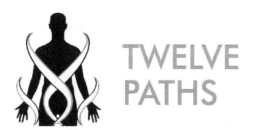

or
Search "@inspiringleaderscollective" on YouTube or Facebook

For loads of free articles, PDF guides, and more related to health, fitness, motivation, and success.

REFERENCES

Shawn Stevenson

1. Stevenson, Shawn. 2016. *Sleep Smarter: 21 Essential Strategies to Sleep Your Way to a Better Body, Better Health, and Bigger Success*. Rodale Books, 240.
2. Vium, Niels. "132 w/ Shawn Stevenson: Better Relationships, Sleep Quality, Nutrition and Exercise". *Mindcast (Podcast)*. Oct 3, 2019. https://soundcloud.com/user-444876921/mindcast-132-w-shawn-stevenson-better-relationships-sleep-quality-nutrition-and-exercise/.
3. *Sleep Smarter*, xviii.
4. *Sleep Smarter*, xix.
5. Dolce, Mike. "Ep. 311 Shawn Stevenson". *The Mike Dolce (Podcast)*. Aug 3, 2020. https://podtail.com/podcast/the-mike-dolce-show/ep-311-shawn-stevenson-full-episode
6. Chappus, Jesse and Marni Wasserman. "027: Shawn Stevenson – Optimize Your Sleep | Don't Underestimate Walking | Blue-Light Blocking". *The Ultimate Health Podcast*. March 23, 2015. https://ultimatehealthpodcast.com/shawn-stevenson/
7. *Sleep Smarter*, 103.
8. *Sleep Smarter*, 13.
9. *Sleep Smarter*, 15.
10. *Sleep Smarter*, 12.
11. *Sleep Smarter*, 76.
12. *Sleep Smarter*, 13.
13. Matthews, Michael. "Shawn Stevenson on How to Get the Best Sleep of Your Life". *Muscle for Life (Podcast)*. May 23, 2015. https://legionathletics.com/shawn-stevenson-podcast/
14. *Sleep Smarter*, xi-xx.
15. *Sleep Smarter*, 2, 5, 89.
16. *Sleep Smarter*, xxi, xxii, xxv, 2-4, 72, 84, 92, 111, 182.

17. *Sleep Smarter*, 159-160.
18. "Shawn Stevenson on How to Get the Best Sleep of Your Life"
19. *Sleep Smarter*, 160.
20. *Sleep Smarter*, 160-161.
21. *Sleep Smarter*, 161-162.
22. *Sleep Smarter*, 9.
23. *Sleep Smarter*, 11-15.
24. *Sleep Smarter*, 19-20
25. *Sleep Smarter*, 25-26.
26. *Sleep Smarter*, 93-99.
27. *Sleep Smarter*, 100.
28. *Sleep Smarter*, 99.
29. *Sleep Smarter*, 100.
30. *Sleep Smarter*, 23.
31. *Sleep Smarter*, 98.
32. *Sleep Smarter*, xxi.
33. Stevenson, Shawn. "TMHS 298: The Sleep & Fat Loss Masterclass". *The Model Health Show (Podcast)*. July 18, 2018. https://themodelhealthshow.com/sleep-fat-loss-masterclass/
34. *Sleep Smarter*, 41.
35. *Sleep Smarter*, 49.
36. *Sleep Smarter*, 6.
37. *Sleep Smarter*, 50.
38. *Sleep Smarter*, 33.
39. *Sleep Smarter*, 121.
40. *Sleep Smarter*, 28-31.
41. *Sleep Smarter*, 34.
42. *Sleep Smarter*, 115-118.
43. *Sleep Smarter*, 122.
44. *Sleep Smarter*, 44-45.
45. *Sleep Smarter*, 47.
46. *Sleep Smarter*, 48.
47. *Sleep Smarter*, 173.
48. *Sleep Smarter*, 35.
49. *Sleep Smarter*, 38.
50. *Sleep Smarter*, 175.
51. *Sleep Smarter*, 92.
52. *Sleep Smarter*, 151.
53. *Sleep Smarter*, 152.
54. *Sleep Smarter*, 151-152.
55. *Sleep Smarter*, 153.
56. *Sleep Smarter*, 154.
57. *Sleep Smarter*, 153.
58. *Sleep Smarter*, 90.

59. *Sleep Smarter*, 82.
60. *Sleep Smarter*, 85.
61. *Sleep Smarter*, 87.
62. *Sleep Smarter*, 81.
63. *Sleep Smarter*, 92.
64. Wells, Katie. "89: Why Sleep Is More Important Than Diet and Exercise Combined with Shawn Stevenson". *Wellness Mama (Podcast)*. July 13, 2017. https://wellnessmama.com/podcast/shawn-stevenson/
65. Howes, Lewis. "896 The Science of Sleep for Ultimate Success with Shawn Stevenson". *The School of Greatness (Podcast)*. Jan 1, 2020. https://podbay.fm/p/the-school-of-greatness/e/1577855053
66. "027: Shawn Stevenson – Optimize Your Sleep | Don't Underestimate Walking | Blue-Light Blocking"
67. *Sleep Smarter*, 90.
68. *Sleep Smarter*, 184-188.
69. *Sleep Smarter*, 53.
70. *Sleep Smarter*, 62.
71. *Sleep Smarter*, 108.
72. *Sleep Smarter*, 56-57.
73. *Sleep Smarter*, 58-59.
74. *Sleep Smarter*, 58.
75. *Sleep Smarter*, 61.
76. *Sleep Smarter*, 60-61.
77. "896 The Science of Sleep for Ultimate Success with Shawn Stevenson".
78. *Sleep Smarter*, 105.
79. *Sleep Smarter*, 107.
80. *Sleep Smarter*, 105-107.
81. Stevenson, Shawn. "TMHS 317: The Heart Masterclass: Blood Pressure, Blood Sugar, & 4 Steps To Perfect Heart Health". *The Model Health Show (Podcast)*. Nov 4, 2018. https://themodelhealthshow.com/heart-health/
82. *Sleep Smarter*, 114.
83. Stevenson, Shawn. "TMHS 358: Truth About Water Supply & How Water Controls Your Health". *The Model Health Show (Podcast)*. June 25, 2019. https://themodelhealthshow.com/truth-water-supply/
84. Stevenson, Shawn. "TMHS 73: Hydration & Water Masterclass – Best Water Filter, Best Bottled Water & Critical Water Facts". *The Model Health Show (Podcast)*. Oct 15, 2014. https://themodelhealthshow.com/best-water-filter-best-bottled-water/
85. *Sleep Smarter*, 145.
86. *Sleep Smarter*, 136-138, 145-146.
87. *Sleep Smarter*, 149.
88. Bilyeu, Tom. "Why Sleep Is More Important Than Diet - Shawn Stevenson on Health Theory". *Impact Theory (Podcast)*. Nov 12, 2018. https://themodelhealthshow.com/best-water-filter-best-bottled-water/

89. "132 w/ Shawn Stevenson: Better Relationships, Sleep Quality, Nutrition and Exercise"
90. *Sleep Smarter*, 178.
91. *Sleep Smarter*, 99.
92. *Sleep Smarter*, 73.
93. *Sleep Smarter*, 69.
94. "Shawn Stevenson on How to Get the Best Sleep of Your Life"
95. *Sleep Smarter*, 148.
96. Michler, Ryan. "039: Living A Healthy Life With Shawn Stevenson". *Order of Man (Podcast)*. Dec 15, 2015. https://www.orderofman.com/healthy-life-with-shawn-stevenson/
97. *Sleep Smarter*, xvi.
98. *Sleep Smarter*, xxiii.
99. *Sleep Smarter*, 10.
100. *Sleep Smarter*, 16.
101. *Sleep Smarter*, 17.
102. *Sleep Smarter*, 34.
103. *Sleep Smarter*, 45.
104. *Sleep Smarter*, 65-66.
105. *Sleep Smarter*, 66.
106. *Sleep Smarter*, 66.
107. *Sleep Smarter*, 66-67.
108. *Sleep Smarter*, 75.
109. *Sleep Smarter*, 76.
110. *Sleep Smarter*, 77.
111. *Sleep Smarter*, 79.
112. *Sleep Smarter*, 80.
113. *Sleep Smarter*, 88.
114. *Sleep Smarter*, 88.
115. *Sleep Smarter*, 91.
116. *Sleep Smarter*, 91.
117. *Sleep Smarter*, 101-102.
118. *Sleep Smarter*, 109.
119. *Sleep Smarter*, 112.
120. *Sleep Smarter*, 112.
121. *Sleep Smarter*, 113.
122. *Sleep Smarter*, 116.
123. *Sleep Smarter*, 117.
124. *Sleep Smarter*, 119.
125. *Sleep Smarter*, 119.
126. *Sleep Smarter*, 124-128.
127. *Sleep Smarter*, 130-131.
128. *Sleep Smarter*, 145-146.
129. *Sleep Smarter*, 146.

130. *Sleep Smarter*, 154.
131. *Sleep Smarter*, 155.
132. *Sleep Smarter*, 162.
133. *Sleep Smarter*, 165-166.
134. *Sleep Smarter*, 170-171.
135. *Sleep Smarter*, 175.
136. *Sleep Smarter*, 176.
137. The Model Health Show. 2020. "Here's 2 Quick Tips to Teach Your Body to Burn More Fat." https://themodelhealthshow. com/2-quick-tips-to-teach-your-body-to-burn-more-fat/.
138. The Model Health Show. 2020. "Colon Cancer, Constipation Relief & Proper Pooping." https://themodelhealthshow.com/ colon-cancer-constipation-relief/.
139. Stevenson, Shawn. "TMHS 16: 9 Tips for Eating Healthy on a Budget & What Does "Healthy" Mean Anyway?". *The Model Health Show (Podcast)*. Sept 5, 2013. https://themodelhealthshow.com/ tips-eating-healthy-budget/
140. Stevenson, Shawn. "TMHS 176: 5 Keys To An Amazing Relationship - With Anne Stevenson". *The Model Health Show (Podcast)*. Sept 20, 2016. https://themodelhealthshow.com/5-keys-to-an-amazing-relationship/
141. "TMHS 298: The Sleep & Fat Loss Masterclass"
142. "TMHS 274: How to Quickly Recover from Sleep Deprivation".
143. "TMHS 274: How to Quickly Recover from Sleep Deprivation".
144. "The Heart Masterclass: Blood Pressure, Blood Sugar, & 4 Steps To Perfect Heart Health".
145. Mylett, Ed. "Shawn Stevenson - How to Sleep Smarter". *The Ed Mylett Show (Podcast)*. April 26, 2018. https://luminarypodcasts.com/listen/ ed-mylett-047/ed-mylett-show/shawn-stevenson-how-to-sleep-smart-er/04fb4ab2-a5a8-47d3-93d5-1d7d60736169
146. "132 w/ Shawn Stevenson: Better Relationships, Sleep Quality, Nutrition and Exercise"
147. "89: Why Sleep Is More Important Than Diet and Exercise Combined with Shawn Stevenson"
148. "896 The Science of Sleep for Ultimate Success with Shawn Stevenson".
149. Marcus, Aubrey. "Masking The Real Health Crisis with Shawn Stevenson - AMP #276". *Aubrey Marcus Podcast*. Sept 30, 2020. https://www.aubreymarcus.com/blogs/aubrey-marcus-podcast/ masking-the-real-health-crisis-with-shawn-stevenson-amp-276
150. Di Stefano, Sal, Adam Schafer & Justin Andrews. "355: Shawn Stevenson- Sleep Expert & Bestselling Author". *Mind Pump (Podcast)*. Aug 28, 2016. https://www.iheart. com/podcast/269-mind-pump-raw-fitness-trut-30917636/ episode/355-shawn-stevenson-sleep-expert-30917940/

Dr. Steven Gundry

1. Gundry, Steven R. 2009. *Dr. Gundry's Diet Evolution: Turn Off the Genes That Are Killing You and Your Waistline.* Harmony, 131.
2. Community of Holistic Living. 2017. "Dr. Steven Gundry M.D. World Renown Hear Surgeon Leaves Profession to Create a Better Solution - Holobiotics." https://cohlinc.com/2017/04/06/dr-steven-gundry-md-world-renown-heart-surgeon-leaves-profession-to-create-a-better-solution-holobiotics/
3. Gundry, Steven R. "About Gundry MD." 2020. https://gundrymd.com/gundry-md/
4. Pakulski, Ben. "53 - Rethinking Everything You Knew About A "Healthy Diet " with Dr. Steven Gundry". *The Muscle Expert Podcast.* Oct 18, 2017. https://www.muscleintelligence.com/gundry/
5. Gundry, Steven R. 2017. *The Plant Paradox: The Hidden Dangers in "Healthy" Foods That Cause Disease and Weight Gain.* 1st ed. Harper Wave, 53-54.
6. *Diet Evolution,* 58-70.
7. *Diet Evolution,* 115.
8. *Diet Evolution,* 22.
9. *Diet Evolution,* 24.
10. *Diet Evolution,* 24.
11. Miles, John R. 2019. "Improving Gut Health Through Diet – A Bold Interview with Dr. Steven R. Gundry." *Bold Business.* https://www.boldbusiness.com/health/steve-gundry-interview-gut-health-importance/. drgundry.com/philosophy
12. Gundry, Steven R. 2020. "Philosophy - Dr Gundry." https://drgundry.com/philosophy/.
13. Russo, Mitch. "027: Dr. Steven Gundry on Why Everything You Know About Diets Are Wrong". *Your First Thousand Clients (Podcast).* Sept 11, 2017. https://mitchrusso.com/027-dr-steven-gundry-everything-know-diets-wrong/
14. Fussman, Cal. "Dr. Steven Gundry: Following Your Purpose". *Big Questions with Cal Fussman (Podcast).* April 2, 2019. https://www.calfussman.com/podcasts/2019/4/2/dr-steven-gundry-following-your-purpose
15. Fishbein, Sami and Aleen Kuperman. "There's Nothing Sexy About A Leaky Gut Ft. Dr. Steven Gundry". *Diet Starts Tomorrow (Podcast).* Aug 12, 2018. https://podtail.com/en/podcast/diet-starts-tomorrow/there-s-nothing-sexy-about-a-leaky-gut-ft-dr-steve/
16. "Dr. Steven Gundry: Following Your Purpose".
17. *Plant Paradox,* 4.
18. Howes, Lewis. "Die Young at An Old Age". *School of Greatness (Podcast).* March 18, 2019. https://lewishowes.com/podcast/how-to-live-a-long-life-with-dr-steven-gundry/

19. *Plant Paradox*, 33-37.
20. *Plant Paradox*, 34.
21. *Plant Paradox*, 68-70.
22. *Plant Paradox*, 249.
23. *Plant Paradox*, 182-183.
24. *Plant Paradox*, 50.
25. *Diet Evolution*, 64.
26. *Plant Paradox*, 237.
27. *Diet Evolution*, 71-72.
28. *Plant Paradox*, 189-197.
29. *Diet Evolution*, 133.
30. *Diet Evolution*, 127-148.
31. *Plant Paradox*, 198-228.
32. *Plant Paradox*, 240.
33. *Diet Evolution*, 149-160.
34. *Plant Paradox*, 229-248.
35. *Diet Evolution*, 163.
36. Longo, Valter D., and Mark P. Mattson. 2014. "Fasting: Molecular Mechanisms and Clinical Applications." *Cell Metabolism* 19 (2): 181–92. doi:10.1016/j.cmet.2013.12.008.
37. Longo, Valter D., Adam Antebi, Andrzej Bartke, Nir Barzilai, Holly M. Brown-Borg, Calogero Caruso, Tyler J. Curiel, et al. 2015. "Interventions to Slow Aging in Humans: Are We Ready?" *Aging Cell* 14 (4): 497–510. doi:10.1111/acel.12338.
38. Gundry, Steven R. 2018. "Valter Longo Interview – Transcript." https://drgundry.com/valter-longo-interview-transcript/.
39. *Plant Paradox*, 244.
40. Orlich, Michael J, Pramil N Singh, Joan Sabaté, Karen Jaceldo-Siegl, Jing Fan, Synnove Knutsen, W. Lawrence Beeson, and Gary E. Fraser. 2013. "Vegetarian Dietary Patterns and Mortality in Adventist Health Study 2." *JAMA Internal Medicine* 173 (13): 1230–38. doi:10.1001/jamainternmed.2013.6473.
41. Gundry, Steven R. 2018. "Abstract P238: Remission/Cure of Autoimmune Diseases by a Lectin Limited Diet Supplemented With Probiotics, Prebiotics, and Polyphenols." *Circulation* 137 (1). https://www.ahajournals.org/doi/abs/10.1161/circ.137.suppl_1.p238.
42. *Plant Paradox*, 247.
43. Gundry MD Team. 2017. "What Is the Best Olive Oil for Maximum Health Benefits?" https://gundrymd.com/best-olive-oil/.
44. *Plant Paradox*, 201-204.
45. *Plant Paradox*, 180-181.
46. *Plant Paradox*, 113-114.
47. *Plant Paradox*, 275.
48. *Diet Evolution*, 106-107, 110-111.

49.   *Diet Evolution*, 33.
50.   *Diet Evolution*, 47.
51.   *Diet Evolution*, 80.
52.   Gundry, Steven R. "047: Carnivore Diet: Crazy delicious, or just plain crazy?". *The Dr. Gundry Podcast.* July 8, 2019. https://drgundry.com/carnivore-diet/
53.   *Diet Evolution*, 81.
54.   *Plant Paradox*, 215.
55.   *Diet Evolution*, 132.
56.   Gundry, Steven R. "021: Is Your Dog The Best Medicine? | Tamar Geller". *The Dr. Gundry Podcast.* Jan 14, 2019. https://drgundry.com/021-is-your-dog-the-best-medicine-tamar-geller/
57.   *Diet Evolution*, 126.
58.   *Diet Evolution*, 120.
59.   Sleep Smarter, xvi.
60.   Gundry, Steven R., and Heather Moday. 2020. "Foods High in Lectins: What To Avoid To Heal Your Gut." *Mindbodygreen.* https://www.mindbodygreen.com/articles/foods-high-in-lectins.
61.   *Diet Evolution*, 144.
62.   *Diet Evolution*, 124.
63.   *Diet Evolution*, 93.

Ben Greenfield

1.   Greenfield, Ben. "Can you Hack Your Biological Age? | Ben Greenfield." *YouTube.* July 26, 2018. https://www.youtube.com/watch?v=p7ccaKmoSfM
2.   "Personal Trainer of the Year." 2020. *National Strength and Conditioning Association.* https://www.nsca.com/membership/awards/annual-awards/pro-coach-of-year4/.
3.   The Greatist Team. 2014. "The 100 Most Influential People in Health and Fitness 2013." *Greatist.* https://greatist.com/discover/most-influential-health-fitness-people-2013.
4.   The Greatist Team. 2015. "The 100 Most Influential People in Health and Fitness 2014." *Greatist.* https://greatist.com/live/most-influential-health-fitness-people-2014
5.   Greenfield, Ben. "About Ben Greenfield." 2017. *Ben Greenfield Fitness.* https://bengreenfieldfitness.com/ben-greenfield/.
6.   Greenfield, Ben. 2014. *Beyond Training: Mastering Endurance, Health & Life.* Victory Belt Publishing, 145.
7.   *Beyond Training*, 56.
8.   *Beyond Training*, 21-27.
9.   *Beyond Training*, 24.

10. *Beyond Training*, 27.
11. *Beyond Training*, 288.
12. *Beyond Training*, 289.
13. Volek, Jeff S., Daniel J. Freidenreich, Catherine Saenz, Laura J. Kunces, Brent C. Creighton, Jenna M. Bartley, Patrick M. Davitt, et al. 2016. "Metabolic Characteristics of Keto-Adapted Ultra-Endurance Runners." *Metabolism*: Clinical and Experimental 65 (3): 100–110. doi:10.1016/j.metabol.2015.10.028.
14. Greenfield, Ben. 2016. "My Exact Evening Routine Unveiled Step-By-Step (Feel Free to Copy, Modify or Comment)." *Ben Greenfield Fitness*. https://bengreenfieldfitness.com/article/lifestyle-articles/ben-greenfields-evening-routine/
15. Greenfield, Ben. 2012. "How I Ate A High Fat Diet, Pooped 8 Pounds, And Then Won A Sprint Triathlon." *Ben Greenfield Fitness*. https://bengreenfieldfitness.com/article/nutrition-articles/why-you-should-squat-to-poop/.
16. Greenfield, Ben. 2014. "Rewriting The Fat Burning Textbook – Part 1: Why You've Been Lied To About Carbs And How To Turn Yourself Into A Fat Burning Machine." *Ben Greenfield Fitness*. https://bengreenfieldfitness.com/article/low-carb-ketogenic-diet-articles/how-much-fat-can-you-burn/.
17. *Beyond Training*, 318-319.
18. "Rewriting The Fat Burning Textbook – Part 1: Why You've Been Lied To About Carbs And How To Turn Yourself Into A Fat Burning Machine."
19. Greenfield, Ben. 2011. "10 Ways To Do A Low Carbohydrate Diet The Right Way." *Ben Greenfield Fitness*. https://bengreenfieldfitness.com/article/low-carb-ketogenic-diet-articles/10-ways-to-do-a-low-carbohydrate-diet-the-right-way/.
20. *Beyond Training*, 290.
21. Greenfield, Ben. 2011. "The Hidden Dangers Of A Low Carbohydrate Diet." *Ben Greenfield Fitness*. https://bengreenfieldfitness.com/article/low-carb-ketogenic-diet-articles/the-hidden-dangers-of-a-low-carbohydrate-diet/.
22. Greenfield, Ben. 2012. "7 Supplements That Help You Perform Better On A Low Carbohydrate Diet." *Ben Greenfield Fitness*. https://bengreenfieldfitness.com/article/low-carb-ketogenic-diet-articles/low-carb-diet-supplements/.
23. Chek, Paul. "Episode 10 - Ben Greenfield - Biohacking, A Deeper Look." *Living 4D with Paul Chek (Podcast)*. Feb 6, 2019. https://www.youtube.com/watch?v=VQXnxLsO6Tg
24. *Beyond Training*, 230-231.
25. *Beyond Training*, 232-233.
26. *Beyond Training*, 92.

27. Greenfield, Ben. "Episode 10 - Ben Greenfield - Biohacking, A Deeper Look 383: How To Maximize Stem Cell Health, Why Branched Chain Amino Acids Don't Work, How To Get A Better Score On A VO2 Max Test & Much More!" *Ben Greenfield Fitness (Podcast)*. March 29, 2018. https://bengreenfieldfitness.com/podcast/383-how-to-maximize-stem-cell-health-why-branched-chain-amino-acids-dont-work-how-to-get-a-better-score-on-a-vo2-max-test-much-more/

28. *Beyond Training*, 153.

29. Divine, Mark. "Ben Greenfield talks to Mark about training and biohacking." *Unbeatable Mind Podcast with Mark Divine*. Nov 2, 2016. https://unbeatablemind.com/ben-greenfield/

30. *Beyond Training*, 79.

31. Greenfield, Ben. 2015. "Ten Scientifically Proven Reasons I Am Addicted To A Daily Sauna." *Ben Greenfield Fitness*. https://bengreenfieldfitness.com/article/biohacking-articles/science-of-sauna/.

32. Wachob, Jason. "189: How to hack your health (eating, sleeping & moving) with Ben Greenfield". *The Mindbodygreen Podcast*. Feb 21, 2020. https://www.stitcher.com/show/the-mindbodygreen-podcast/episode/189-how-to-hack-your-health-eating-sleeping-moving-with-ben-greenfield-67503954

33. Greenfield, Ben. "How You Can Use Cold Thermogenesis To Perform Like Lance Armstrong And Michael Phelps." *Ben Greenfield Fitness (Podcast)*. June 15, 2012. https://bengreenfieldfitness.com/podcast/biohacking-podcasts/cold-thermogenesis-how-to/

34. *Beyond Training*, 74.

35. Rogen, Joe. "#1069 - Ben Greenfield". *The Joe Rogan Experience (Podcast)*. Jan 29, 2018. https://www.podchaser.com/podcasts/the-joe-rogan-experience-10829/episodes/1069-ben-greenfield-25112955

36. *Beyond Training*, 383.

37. Greenfield, Ben. "How To Reverse The Damage From Cell Phone Radiation, Hidden Sources Of EMF, The Best Way To Measure Your EMF Exposure & Much More With Dr. Joseph Mercola!" *Ben Greenfield Fitness (Podcast)*. Feb 3, 2018. https://bengreenfieldfitness.com/podcast/lifestyle-podcasts/dr-mercola-emf-recommendations/

38. Vroman, Jon. "The Ultimate Unschooling Adventure with Ben Greenfield". *Front Row Dads (Podcast)*. June 11, 2019. https://frontrowdads.com/ben-greenfield/

39. "Can you Hack Your Biological Age? | Ben Greenfield."

40. Greenfield, Ben. 2013. "Is That Grain Of Salt Really Killing Your Insides?" *Ben Greenfield Fitness*. https://bengreenfieldfitness.com/article/nutrition-articles/grain-salt-really-killing-insides/.

41. *Beyond Training*, 96, 454-455.

42. Greenfield, Ben. 2018. "How To Hack Your Workplace For Enhanced Productivity, Less Muscle Pain, Better Focus & More."

Ben Greenfield Fitness. https://bengreenfieldfitness.com/article/ben-greenfields-home-office-setup/.

43. *Beyond Training,* 207.
44. *Beyond Training,* 92-93.
45. *Beyond Training,* 105.
46. *Beyond Training,* 106.
47. *Beyond Training,* 107.
48. Greenfield, Ben. 2017. "The Misunderstood, Misused Darlings Of The Supplement Industry (& How *Not* To Waste Your Money Or Damage Your Health With Them)." *Ben Greenfield Fitness.* https://bengreenfieldfitness.com/article/supplements-articles/how-to-use-amino-acids-supplements/
49. *Beyond Training,* 108.
50. *Beyond Training,* 187.
51. "189: How to hack your health (eating, sleeping & moving) with Ben Greenfield"
52. Greenfield, Ben. "Smart Drugs, Nootropics, Microdosing With Psychedelics, Enhancing Deep Sleep, Rites Of Passage & Much More With Kyle Kingsbury Of Onnit." *Ben Greenfield Fitness (Podcast).* May 11, 2019. https://bengreenfieldfitness.com/podcast/biohacking-podcasts/enhance-deep-sleep/
53. *Beyond Training,* 93.
54. Greenfield, Ben. "CBD & Cannabis Special Episode: How CBD Affects Hormones, Fat Loss, Athletic Performance, Sleep, Recovery & Much More." *Ben Greenfield Fitness (Podcast).* May 31, 2019. https://bengreenfieldfitness.com/podcast/brain-podcasts/cbd-athletes-benefits/
55. *Beyond Training,* 105.
56. *Beyond Training,* 115.
57. *Beyond Training,* 127.
58. *Beyond Training,* 135-136.
59. *Beyond Training,* 154.
60. *Beyond Training,* 48.
61. *Beyond Training,* 220.
62. *Beyond Training,* 257.
63. Greenfield, Ben. 2019. "The 11 Best Biomarkers To Track If You Want To Live A Long Time & Feel Good Doing It." *Ben Greenfield Fitness.* https://bengreenfieldfitness.com/article/self-quantification-articles/top-lab-tests/.
64. *Beyond Training,* 398.
65. *Beyond Training,* 222.
66. Greenfield, Ben. 2012. *Get-Fit Guy's Guide to Achieving Your Ideal Body: A Workout Plan for Your Unique Shape (Quick & Dirty Tips).* St. Martin's Griffin, 135-136.
67. *Beyond Training,* 214-215.
68. *Beyond Training,* 305, 442.

69. Greenfield, Ben. "Ben Greenfield's Top Anti-Aging Tactics: Basic & Ancestral Strategies To Enhance Longevity." *Ben Greenfield Fitness (Podcast)*. June 6, 2019. https://bengreenfieldfitness.com/podcast/anti-aging-podcasts/anti-aging-tips-2/

Michael Matthews

1. Matthews, Michael. 2019. *Bigger Leaner Stronger: The Simple Science of Building the Ultimate Male Body.* 3rd ed. Oculus Publishers, 31.
2. Barnard, Tom. "Dayna Lee-Baggley and Michael Matthews - #1654-2." Produced by 92 KQRS. *The Tom Barnard Show (Podcast).* July 24, 2019. https://omny.fm/shows/the-tom-barnard-show/dayna-lee-baggley-and-michael-matthews-1654-2.
3. *Bigger Leaner Stronger,* 59.
4. *Bigger Leaner Stronger,* 38.
5. *Bigger Leaner Stronger,* 93.
6. *Bigger Leaner Stronger,* 60.
7. *Bigger Leaner Stronger,* 176-181.
8. Matthews, Michael. 2019. *Thinner Leaner Stronger: The Simple Science of Building the Ultimate Female Body.* 3rd ed. Occulus Publishers, 175-179.
9. *Bigger Leaner Stronger,* 179.
10. Matthews, Michael, and Brian Grant. 2020. "The Easiest Way to Know if You Should Cut or Bulk." *Legion.* https://legionathletics.com/cut-or-bulk/.
11. *Bigger Leaner Stronger,* 254.
12. *Bigger Leaner Stronger,* 97.
13. *Bigger Leaner Stronger,* 102.
14. *Bigger Leaner Stronger,* 97.
15. *Bigger Leaner Stronger,* 163.
16. *Bigger Leaner Stronger,* 176-181.
17. *Thinner Leaner Stronger,* 175-178.
18. *Bigger Leaner Stronger,* 273.
19. Matthews, Michael. "Mark Rippetoe on Training for Strength vs. "Aesthetics" Pt 1". *Muscle for Life with Michael Matthews (Podcast).* July 15, 2016. https://legionathletics.com/mark-rippetoe-interview-part-1/.
20. *Bigger Leaner Stronger,* 229.
21. *Bigger Leaner Stronger,* 81.
22. *Bigger Leaner Stronger,* 237-238.
23. *Bigger Leaner Stronger,* 357.
24. *Bigger Leaner Stronger,* 356.
25. *Bigger Leaner Stronger,* 230-234.

26. Matthews, Michael. "What Makes a Good Pre Workout Supplement?". *Muscle for Life with Michael Matthews (Podcast)*. May 25, 2020. https://legionathletics.com/pre-workout-supplement/.
27. *Bigger Leaner Stronger*, 315.
28. *Bigger Leaner Stronger*, 317.
29. "What Makes a Good Pre Workout Supplement?"
30. Matthews, Michael, and Brian Grant. 2020. "Everything You Need to Know About Pre-Workout Supplements." *Legion*. https://legionathletics.com/pre-workout-supplements/.
31. Matthews, Michael. 2020. "This Is Everything You Need to Know About Post-Workout Nutrition." *Legion*. https://legionathletics.com/everything-need-know-post-workout-nutrition/.
32. What Makes a Good Pre Workout Supplement?"
33. *Bigger Leaner Stronger*, 305.
34. *Bigger Leaner Stronger*, 304-315.
35. Matthews, Michael. 2018. *The Little Black Book of Workout Motivation*. 1st ed. Oculus Publishers, 24.
36. *The Little Black Book of Workout Motivation*, 37.
37. *The Little Black Book of Workout Motivation*, 53.
38. *The Little Black Book of Workout Motivation*, 93.
39. *The Little Black Book of Workout Motivation*, 150.
40. *The Little Black Book of Workout Motivation*, 164.
41. *The Little Black Book of Workout Motivation*, 153.
42. *The Little Black Book of Workout Motivation*, 51.
43. *The Little Black Book of Workout Motivation*, 98-99.
44. Matthews, Michael. "Ru Anderson on How to Master Your Habits (and Thus Your Life)". *Muscle for Life with Michael Matthews (Podcast)*. Mar 4, 2016. https://legionathletics.com/ru-anderson-interview/.
45. Harb, Mitch. "Ep 182: Michael Matthews- How to Get Bigger, Leaner, Stronger Without Living In The Gym". *The Easy Wins Podcast*. July 29, 2019. https://poddtoppen.se/podcast/1290900322/the-easy-wins-podcast/ep-182-mike-matthews-how-to-get-bigger-leaner-stronger-without-living-in-the-gym.
46. *Bigger Leaner Stronger*, 70.
47. *Bigger Leaner Stronger*, 84.
48. *Bigger Leaner Stronger*, 86.
49. *Bigger Leaner Stronger*, 98-99.
50. *Bigger Leaner Stronger*, 109.
51. *Bigger Leaner Stronger*, 123.
52. *Bigger Leaner Stronger*, 124.
53. *Bigger Leaner Stronger*, 125.
54. *Bigger Leaner Stronger*, 126.
55. *Bigger Leaner Stronger*, 128.
56. *Bigger Leaner Stronger*, 129.

57.   *Bigger Leaner Stronger*, 133.
58.   *Bigger Leaner Stronger*, 135.
59.   *Bigger Leaner Stronger*, 142.
60.   *Bigger Leaner Stronger*, 206.
61.   *Bigger Leaner Stronger*, 187.
62.   *Bigger Leaner Stronger*, 190.
63.   *Bigger Leaner Stronger*, 216.
64.   *Bigger Leaner Stronger*, 251.
65.   *Bigger Leaner Stronger*, 253.
66.   *Bigger Leaner Stronger*, 270.
67.   *Bigger Leaner Stronger*, 271.
68.   *Bigger Leaner Stronger*, 189.
69.   *Bigger Leaner Stronger*, 311.
70.   *Bigger Leaner Stronger*, 313.
71.   *Bigger Leaner Stronger*, 340.
72.   *Bigger Leaner Stronger*, 349.
73.   *Bigger Leaner Stronger*, 381.
74.   *Bigger Leaner Stronger*, 385.
75.   *Bigger Leaner Stronger*, 384-385.
76.   *Bigger Leaner Stronger*, 425.
77.   *The Little Black Book of Workout Motivation*, 100.
78.   *The Little Black Book of Workout Motivation*, 113.
79.   *The Little Black Book of Workout Motivation*, 116.
80.   *The Little Black Book of Workout Motivation*, 184.
81.   *The Little Black Book of Workout Motivation*, 192.
82.   *The Little Black Book of Workout Motivation*, 202.
83.   Matthews, Michael. 2020. "How Much Water Should I Drink? A Simple & Science-Based Answer." *Legion*. https://legionathletics.com/how-much-water-should-i-drink/.
84.   Matthews, Michael. "How Much Cardio You Should Do (and How Much Is Too Much)?". *Muscle for Life with Michael Matthews (Podcast)*. April 3, 2019. https://legionathletics.com/how-much-cardio-podcast/
85.   *Bigger Leaner Stronger*, 248.
86.   *Bigger Leaner Stronger*, 250.
87.   *Bigger Leaner Stronger*, 427.
88.   *Bigger Leaner Stronger*, 98-99.
89.   Matthews, Michael. 2020. "7 Proven Ways to Sleep Better Than Ever Before." *Legion*. https://legionathletics.com/how-to-sleep-better/.
90.   *Bigger Leaner Stronger*, 255.
91.   Matthews, Michael, and Brian Grant. 2020. "Is Milk Bad For You? What 30 Studies Have to Say." *Legion*. https://legionathletics.com/is-milk-bad-for-you/.
92.   Matthews, Michael. "My Interview with Lacey Dunn on Starting a Business, Book Publishing, and More". *Muscle for Life with Michael*

Matthews (Podcast). May 25, 2020. https://legionathletics.com/
lacey-dunn-interview/.

93. *Bigger Leaner Stronger,* 320.
94. *Bigger Leaner Stronger,* 401.
95. *The Little Black Book of Workout Motivation*, 64.
96. *Bigger Leaner Stronger,* 93.

Dr. Cate Shanahan

1.   Shanahan, Catherine. 2020. *The Fatburn Fix: Boost Energy, End Hunger,
     and Lose Weight by Using Body Fat for Fuel Hardcover.* 1st ed. Flatiron
     Books, 333.
2.   Kearns, Brad. "Dr. Cate Shanahan: How to Become Can-
     cer-Proof!" *The B.rad Podcast.* Nov 26, 2019. https://www.
     stitcher.com/show/get-over-yourself-podcast/episode/
     dr-cate-shanahan-how-to-become-cancer-proof-65567605
3.   Shanahan, Catherine, and Luke Shanahan. 2018. *Deep Nutrition: Why
     Your Genes Need Traditional Food.* Flatiron Books, 10.
4.   "An Interview with Dr. Cate Shanahan." 2013. *Lakers.com* https://www.
     nba.com/lakers/training_staff/131203_interview_shanahan.
5.   Jacobs, Richard. "Deep Thoughts About Nutrition – Dr.
     Cate Shanahan – drcate.com." *Finding Genius Podcast.* Oct
     22, 2019. https://www.findinggeniuspodcast.com/podcasts/
     deep-thoughts-about-nutrition-dr-cate-shanahan-drcate-com/
6.   Starrett, Kelly and Juliet Starrett. "S1EP8: Dr. Cate Sha-
     nahan". *The Ready State (Podcast).* Jan 15, 2018. https://
     www.stitcher.com/show/get-over-yourself-podcast/episode/
     dr-cate-shanahan-how-to-become-cancer-proof-65567605
7.   Whittel, Naomi. "The Real Skinny on Fat The Truth About Weight
     Loss Episode 1." *YouTube.* March 2, 2018. https://www.youtube.com/
     watch?v=CdoSSaKjv7A&feature=emb_title.
8.   *Deep Nutrition,* 126.
9.   *Deep Nutrition,* 144.
10. *Deep Nutrition,* 131.
11. *Deep Nutrition,* 163.
12. *Deep Nutrition,* 167.
13. *Deep Nutrition,* 187.
14. "What & Where the Doctors Eat — Dr. Cate Shana-
     han." 2017. *Re-Find Health.* https://re-findhealth.com/post/
     where-the-doctors-eat-cate-shanahan/.
15. Shanahan, Catherine. 2017. "List of Good Fats and Oils versus Bad." *Dr
     Cate.* https://drcate.com/list-of-good-fats-and-oils-versus-bad/.
16. *Deep Nutrition,* 210-224.

17. *Deep Nutrition*, 229-231.
18. *Deep Nutrition*, 336.
19. *Deep Nutrition*, 92.
20. *Deep Nutrition*, 426.
21. *Deep Nutrition*, 44.
22. *Deep Nutrition*, xvii.
23. Stevenson, Shawn. "TMHS 297: The Truth About Collagen, Genetic Plasticity, & Sugar Bombs - With Guest Dr. Cate Shanahan". *The Model Health Show (Podcast)*. July 10, 2018. https://themodelhealthshow.com/cate-shanahan/
24. *Deep Nutrition*, 244.
25. *Deep Nutrition*, 303.
26. James, Abel. "Dr. Cate Shanahan: Why Kobe Bryant Drinks Bone Broth." *Fat-Burning Man (Podcast)*. Jan 20, 2017. https://fatburningman.com/dr-cate-shanahan-why-kobe-bryant-drinks-bone-broth/
27. *Deep Nutrition*, 323.
28. *Deep Nutrition*, 255-256.
29. *Deep Nutrition*, 405.
30. *Deep Nutrition*, 260-261.
31. Greenfield, Ben "4 Ways To Eat Yourself Beautiful: Meat On The Bone, Fermented & Sprouted Foods, Organ Meats, Deep Nutrition & More With Dr. Cate Shanahan." *Ben Greenfield Fitness (Podcast)*. March 29, 2017. https://bengreenfieldfitness.com/podcast/nutrition-podcasts/deep-nutrition-book-2/
32. *Deep Nutrition*, 265.
33. "4 Ways To Eat Yourself Beautiful: Meat On The Bone, Fermented & Sprouted Foods, Organ Meats, Deep Nutrition & More With Dr. Cate Shanahan."
34. *Deep Nutrition*, 271-272.
35. *Deep Nutrition*, 74.
36. *Deep Nutrition*, 85-86.
37. *Deep Nutrition*, 95-96.
38. *Deep Nutrition*, 20.
39. *Deep Nutrition*, 88.
40. *Deep Nutrition*, 97.
41. *Deep Nutrition*, 162.
42. *Deep Nutrition*, 155.
43. *Deep Nutrition*, 151.
44. Bubbs, Mark "EPISODE 28 - Deep Nutrition: Why Your Genes Need Traditional Foods w/ Dr. Cate Shanahan." *The Performance Nutrition Podcast*. July 13, 2017. https://drbubbs.com/podcastepisodes/2017/7/episode-28-deep-nutrition-why-your-genes-need-traditional-foods-cate-shanahan
45. *Deep Nutrition*, 214-215.

46. *Deep Nutrition*, 145.
47. Kearns, Brad "Setting Things Straight With Dr. Cate Shanahan." *Get Over Yourself (Podcast)*. Sept 3, 2019. https://www.bradkearns.com/2019/09/03/shanahan2/
48. Ambrosini, Melissa "93: The Silent Killer In Your Food With Dr Cate Shanahan." *The Melissa Ambrosini Show (Podcast)*. May 2, 2018. https://melissaambrosini.com/podcast/the-silent-killer-in-your-food-with-dr-cate-shanahan/
49. *Deep Nutrition*, 365.
50. *The Fatburn Fix*, 2.
51. *The Fatburn Fix*, 11.
52. *The Fatburn Fix*, 34-35.
53. *The Fatburn Fix*, 54.
54. *The Fatburn Fix*, 2.
55. *The Fatburn Fix*, 51.
56. *The Fatburn Fix*, 49.
57. *The Fatburn Fix*, 14.
58. *The Fatburn Fix*, 11.
59. *The Fatburn Fix*, 28.
60. *The Fatburn Fix*, 186.
61. *The Fatburn Fix*, 195.
62. *The Fatburn Fix*, 127.
63. *The Fatburn Fix*, 138-139.
64. *The Fatburn Fix*, 202-205.
65. *The Fatburn Fix*, 208.
66. *The Fatburn Fix*, 214-215.
67. *The Fatburn Fix*, 159-161.
68. *The Fatburn Fix*, 151.
69. *The Fatburn Fix*, 189.
70. *The Fatburn Fix*, 225.
71. *The Fatburn Fix*, 228.
72. *The Fatburn Fix*, 123.
73. *The Fatburn Fix*, 119-120.
74. *The Fatburn Fix*, 280.
75. *The Fatburn Fix*, 286-291.
76. *The Fatburn Fix*, 282-284.
77. *The Fatburn Fix*, 245.
78. *The Fatburn Fix*, 255-256.
79. *The Fatburn Fix*, 280.
80. *The Fatburn Fix*, 292.
81. Lenzekes, Brian, Tro Kalayjian, Jason Fung, and Megan Ramos. "Episode 27: Cate Shanahan." *Low Carb MD Podcast*. April 8, 2019. https://lowcarbmd.com/episode-27-cate-shanahan
82. *Deep Nutrition*, 94.

83. *Deep Nutrition*, 21.
84. *Deep Nutrition*, 49.
85. *Deep Nutrition*, 55-57.
86. *Deep Nutrition*, 73.
87. *Deep Nutrition*, 95.
88. *Deep Nutrition*, 96.
89. *Deep Nutrition*, 107.
90. *Deep Nutrition*, 118.
91. *Deep Nutrition*, 139.
92. *Deep Nutrition*, 165-169.
93. *Deep Nutrition*, 167-168.
94. *Deep Nutrition*, 168.
95. *Deep Nutrition*, 184.
96. *Deep Nutrition*, 189-192.
97. *Deep Nutrition*, 198.
98. *Deep Nutrition*, 203.
99. *Deep Nutrition*, 222.
100. *Deep Nutrition*, 249.
101. *Deep Nutrition*, 262-264.
102. *Deep Nutrition*, 282.
103. *Deep Nutrition*, 292.
104. *Deep Nutrition*, 298.
105. *Deep Nutrition*, 311.
106. *Deep Nutrition*, 316.
107. *Deep Nutrition*, 331.
108. *Deep Nutrition*, 333-334.
109. *Deep Nutrition*, 337.
110. *Deep Nutrition*, 374.
111. *Deep Nutrition*, 394.
112. *Deep Nutrition*, 398.
113. *Deep Nutrition*, 408.
114. *Deep Nutrition*, 410-411.
115. *The Fatburn Fix*, 209.
116. *Deep Nutrition*, 412.
117. *Deep Nutrition*, 420-421.
118. Matthews, Michael. "Dr. Cate Shanahan on the Power of "Deep Nutrition"." *Muscle for Life (Podcast)*. July 19, 2017. https://legionathletics.com/dr-cate-shanahan-podcast/
119. *The Fatburn Fix*, 47.
120. *The Fatburn Fix*, 43.
121. *The Fatburn Fix*, 62.
122. *The Fatburn Fix*, 65.
123. *The Fatburn Fix*, 53.
124. *The Fatburn Fix*, 85.

125. *The Fatburn Fix*, 67-69.
126. *The Fatburn Fix*, 87.
127. *The Fatburn Fix*, 88.
128. *The Fatburn Fix*, 115.
129. *The Fatburn Fix*, 256.
130. *The Fatburn Fix*, 122.
131. *The Fatburn Fix*, 216.
132. *The Fatburn Fix*, 217.
133. *The Fatburn Fix*, 222.
134. *The Fatburn Fix*, 230.
135. *The Fatburn Fix*, 235.
136. *The Fatburn Fix*, 249.
137. *The Fatburn Fix*, 273.
138. *The Fatburn Fix*, 314.
139. *The Fatburn Fix*, 316.
140. *The Fatburn Fix*, 323.
141. *The Fatburn Fix*, 95.
142. *The Fatburn Fix*, 99.
143. *The Fatburn Fix*, 103.
144. *The Fatburn Fix*, 100.
145. *Deep Nutrition*, 20.
146. *Deep Nutrition*, 117.
147. *Deep Nutrition*, 232.
148. *Deep Nutrition*, 249.
149. *Deep Nutrition*, 250.
150. *Deep Nutrition*, 300.
151. *Deep Nutrition*, 279.
152. *Deep Nutrition*, 282.
153. *Deep Nutrition*, 284-287.
154. *Deep Nutrition*, 393.

Dr. Kelly Starrett

1. Chewning, Chase. "How to Best Recover from Injuries and Training for the Infinite Game with Kelly Starrett." *Ever Forward Radio (Podcast)*. Oct 31, 2019. https://www.pod-chaser.com/podcasts/ever-forward-radio-431429/episodes/efr-242-how-to-best-recover-fr-47254818

2. "What Is *The Ready State*." 2021. *The Ready State*. https://thereadystate.com/the-trs-difference/#trsteam

3. McKay, Jimmy. "54 – Kelly Starrett on Movement, Performance & Injury." *PT Pintcast (Podcast)*. Feb 9, 2016. https://www.ptpintcast.com/2016/02/09/ep-54/

4.	DeFranco, Joe. "#7 Kelly Starrett Interview." *Joe DeFranco's Industrial Strength Show (Podcast)*. April 16, 2015. https://www.defrancostraining.com/kelly-starrett-interview/

5.	Doyon, Ricky. "Ep.2 Kelly Starrett." *Alpha Brew Podcast*. April 2, 2019. https://www.iheart.com/podcast/256-alpha-brew-podcast-43099687/episode/ep2-kelly-starrett-45014223/

6.	Starrett, Kelly, and Glen Cordoza. 2016. *Deskbound: Standing Up to a Sitting World*. Victory Belt Publishing.

7.	"What Is *the Ready State*."

8.	Pastuch, Sean. "112 - Kelly Starrett - What is Mobility." *The Active Life Podcast*. Dec 10, 2018. https://activelife.libsyn.com/kstarr

9.	"Ep.2 Kelly Starrett."

10.	James, Abel. "Dr. Kelly Starrett: Becoming a Supple Leopard, Hacking Human Movement, and Why YOU Move Like an Ass." Fat-Burning Man (Podcast). July 6, 2018. https://fatburningman.com/dr-kelly-starrett-becoming-a-supple-leopard/

11.	Starrett, Kelly (@thereadystate). "All good models are explanatory, predictive, repeatable. Create a model. Try and break it. Over and over. It should work across scale and cohort. Sport is the lab. Simplify, refine. Create elegance. Then watch the doors get blown off and get back to work. @calstrength @weskitts22." *Twitter*. May 9, 2018. https://twitter.com/thereadystate/status/994329538439012354

12.	Starrett, Kelly, and Glen Cordoza. 2013. *Becoming a Supple Leopard: The Ultimate Guide to Resolving Pain, Preventing Injury, and Optimizing Athletic Performance*. Victory Belt Publishing, 24.

13.	*Becoming a Supple Leopard*, 15.

14.	*Becoming a Supple Leopard*, 55.

15.	*Becoming a Supple Leopard*, 63.

16.	*Becoming a Supple Leopard*, 71.

17.	*Becoming a Supple Leopard*, 91.

18.	*Becoming a Supple Leopard*, 443.

19.	*Becoming a Supple Leopard*, 272.

20.	*Becoming a Supple Leopard*, 53.

21.	*Deskbound*, 294.

22.	*Becoming a Supple Leopard*, 118.

23.	Ferris, Tim. "The Good, The Bad, and The Ugly of CrossFit (#64)." *The Tim Ferriss Show (Podcast). March* 4, 2015. https://tim.blog/2015/03/04/the-good-the-bad-and-the-ugly-of-crossfit/

24.	*Becoming a Supple Leopard*, 282.

25.	*Becoming a Supple Leopard*, 142.

26.	*Becoming a Supple Leopard*, 143.

27.	*Becoming a Supple Leopard*, 145.

28.	*Deskbound*, 230.

29.	*Becoming a Supple Leopard*, 144.

30. *Becoming a Supple Leopard*, 144-151.
31. *Becoming a Supple Leopard*, 471.
32. *Deskbound*, 8-9.
33. "EFR 242: How to Best Recover from Injuries and Training for the Infinite Game with Kelly Starrett."
34. *Deskbound*, 13.
35. *Deskbound*, 17.
36. *Deskbound*, 15.
37. *Deskbound*, 8-9.
38. CreativeLive. "Kelly Starrett on the Importance of Standing Desks in the Workplace." *YouTube.* May 12, 2016. https://www.youtube.com/watch?v=UAeyeEm-4Sk.
39. *Deskbound*, 23.
40. *Deskbound*, 17.
41. *Deskbound*, 10.
42. *Deskbound*, 15.
43. *Deskbound*, 23.
44. *Deskbound*, 11.
45. *Deskbound*, 164.
46. *Deskbound*, 44-47.
47. *Deskbound*, 90-93.
48. *Deskbound*, 138-139.
49. *Deskbound*, 162.
50. *Deskbound*, 180.
51. *Deskbound*, 168.
52. *Deskbound*, 170-178.
53. *Deskbound*, 209.
54. Stevenson, Shawn. "TMHS 281: Boost Performance, Prevent Injuries & Upgrade Your Movement Diet with Dr. Kelly Starrett." *The Model Health Show (Podcast).* April 15, 2018. https://themodelhealthshow.com/movement-diet/
55. Starrett, Kelly and Juliet Starrett. "S3EP6: Dr. Mark Benden." *The Ready State (Podcast).* Dec 7, 2018. https://members.thereadystate.com/mwod_podcast/s3ep6-dr-mark-benden/
56. Asprey, Dave. "Kelly Starrett: Systems Thinking, Movement, & Running." *Bulletproof Radio (Podcast).* Dec 23, 2014. https://daveasprey.com/kelly-starrett-systems-thinking-movement-standards-getting-ready-to-run-156/
57. *Deskbound*, 212.
58. "Kelly Starrett: Systems Thinking, Movement, & Running".
59. *Deskbound*, 210.
60. "TMHS 281: Boost Performance, Prevent Injuries & Upgrade Your Movement Diet with Dr. Kelly Starrett."

61. "Dr. Kelly Starrett: Becoming a Supple Leopard, Hacking Human Movement, and Why YOU Move Like an Ass."
62. *Deskbound*, 12.
63. *Becoming a Supple Leopard*, 39.
64. *Becoming a Supple Leopard*, 47-48.
65. *Becoming a Supple Leopard*, 52.
66. *Becoming a Supple Leopard*, 59.
67. *Becoming a Supple Leopard*, 62.
68. *Becoming a Supple Leopard*, 76.
69. *Becoming a Supple Leopard*, 96.
70. *Becoming a Supple Leopard*, 126-128.
71. *Becoming a Supple Leopard*, 132.
72. *Becoming a Supple Leopard*, 141.
73. *Becoming a Supple Leopard*, 152.
74. *Becoming a Supple Leopard*, 155.
75. *Becoming a Supple Leopard*, 156-157.
76. *Becoming a Supple Leopard*, 164-165.
77. *Becoming a Supple Leopard*, 176.
78. *Becoming a Supple Leopard*, 196.
79. *Becoming a Supple Leopard*, 207.
80. *Becoming a Supple Leopard*, 208.
81. *Becoming a Supple Leopard*, 220.
82. *Becoming a Supple Leopard*, 221.
83. *Becoming a Supple Leopard*, 227.
84. *Becoming a Supple Leopard*, 232.
85. *Becoming a Supple Leopard*, 259.
86. *Becoming a Supple Leopard*, 350.
87. *Becoming a Supple Leopard*, 363.
88. *Becoming a Supple Leopard*, 425.
89. *Deskbound*, 76.
90. *Becoming a Supple Leopard*, 439.
91. *Deskbound*, 25.
92. *Deskbound*, 144.
93. *Deskbound*, 26.
94. *Deskbound*, 25.
95. *Deskbound*, 69.
96. *Deskbound*, 71.
97. *Deskbound*, 91.
98. *Deskbound*, 106.
99. *Deskbound*, 124.
100. *Deskbound*, 143.
101. *Deskbound*, 156.
102. *Deskbound*, 158.
103. *Deskbound*, 181.

104. *Deskbound*, 194.
105. *Deskbound*, 195.
106. *Deskbound*, 200.
107. *Deskbound*, 202.
108. *Deskbound*, 203.
109. *Deskbound*, 209.
110. *Deskbound*, 210.
111. "TMHS 281: Boost Performance, Prevent Injuries & Upgrade Your Movement Diet with Dr. Kelly Starrett."
112. Jones, Dustin. "Kelly Starrett on OLD≠WEAK-Scaling Elite Athletics to Older Adults @*MobilityWOD*." Bulletproof Radio (Podcast). Feb 7, 2017. https://seniorrehab.libsyn.com/srps-2-kelly-starrett-on-oldweak-scaling-elite-athletics-to-older-adults-*mobilitywod*
113. "Kelly Starrett: Systems Thinking, Movement, & Running."
114. Beshara, James. "#23 — Kelly Starrett — Foundational Thinking." *Below the Line (Podcast)*. July 8, 2019. https://anchor.fm/belowtheline/episodes/23--Kelly-Starrett--Foundational-Thinking-e4id6e
115. *Becoming a Supple Leopard*, 35.
116. *Becoming a Supple Leopard*, 131.
117. *Becoming a Supple Leopard*, 129-130.
118. *Deskbound*, 157.
119. *Deskbound*, 211.
120. Matthews, Michael. 2019. *Thinner Leaner Stronger: The Simple Science of Building the Ultimate Female Body*. 3rd ed. Oculus Publishers, 463.
121. *Becoming a Supple Leopard*, 79-81.
122. *Becoming a Supple Leopard*, 83.

CPSIA information can be obtained
at www.ICGtesting.com
Printed in the USA
JSHW022038130521
14722JS00001B/10